# DIET OUT . . . OREGON

The Oregon Dieters Bluebook

JUDITH S. MAJORS

APPLE PRESS
Milwaukie, Oregon

To: The Oregon Affiliate, Inc.
American Diabetes Association, Inc.

May our education programs continue to make life easier for diabetics and persons on special diets — until a cure is found.

Judy


Printed in the United States of America

Library of Congress Catalog Card Number 81-66715

ISBN 0-9602238-4-3

Published by:
Apple Press
5536 S.E. Harlow
Milwaukie, Oregon 97222

Cover Design: Carrie Ann Majors

With much heartfelt thanks:

Restaurant owners and managers: cooperation and sharing
Jack and Carrie: testing and tasting
"Mom": technical assistance
Special "dieters": sharing your needs

# PREFACE . . . .

Diet Out . . . Oregon is designed to make dieting out fun, simple and nutritionally sound for persons on a special diet or with modified dietary needs.

This guide will supply restaurant information on available entrees, method of preparation, portion sizes, substitutions allowed and availability of diet options.

A person on a special diet does not need to be treated differently than other restaurant patrons. Knowing what is available and how it can be prepared make dieting out a pleasure!

Included are sociable spirit ideas – non-alcoholic beverages with honest to goodness bar names. A drink with a name is the same as the rest of the party . . . plain tomato juice sounds like an exception!

It is often wise to call before trying a new restaurant. Things change rapidly in the restaurant business and today's steak house may be tomorrow's deli!

Fast foods are an important factor in our busy lifestyle. Included is caloric and nutritional information on many Oregon fast food chains. National chain information is standard wherever you travel.

Vacationing is easier if you know where and what foods are available. Slip the guide in your suitcase or make reservations ahead and enjoy a diet safe vacation! Many relaxing, tourist perfect places have good diet options.

Enjoy eating out. Stay happy, stay healthy and be diet wise!

## RULES OF THE ROAD . . .

Dieting out can be simple, fun and healthy! Here are a few simple guidelines to make your meal out diet perfect.

1. Know what your meal requirements are so you may order accordingly.

2. Ask how foods are prepared. Most restaurants will broil any entree item if they have the facility.

3. Check to see if fats are added to vegetables, rice, etc. It may often be omitted.

4. Ask about allowable substitutions if something in the meal is not on your diet. Example: vegetables are often substituted for potatoes. (You are paying for the food . . . you might as well have something you can eat!)

5. Request salad dressings, sauces, gravies and potato toppings on the side. You then control the portion.

6. Make reservations if possible to avoid long . . . too hungry . . . waits.

7. Ask for a doggie bag. Take leftovers home to enjoy the next day. Often it is wise to get the doggie bag at the beginning of a meal and slip the over-size portion into it to avoid temptation of "extra" bites. If 4 oz. is all that's on your plate, that's all you'll eat. You enjoy the rest of the meal and won't miss the extra.

8. If special requests are necessary, allow extra time for preparation.

9. Call ahead if there's a question if requests can be handled or to see what is offered.

10. Traveling by air? Request a diabetic or special diet meal at the time of reservation. Airlines are most accomodating.

11. If dessert comes with your meal often fresh fruit may be substituted. Ice cream can occasionally fit into a diet plan. (1/2 cup equals 1 bread and 2 fat exchanges, 160 calories.)

## THE SOCIAL SPIRIT

Alcohol is a source of many "hidden" calories (7 per gram) and is essentially void of other nutrients. Beer and wine contain carbohydrates in addition to the alcohol and all this must be figured into the diet.

Enjoy the spirit of socializing without the "spirits." There are "non-alcoholic" bar beverages that have real names, look like their spirited cousins, taste much like their alcoholic counterpart and fit into a modified diet.

A Greyhound is grapefruit juice and gin. Simply order the Virgin Greyhound and you'll get a glass of grapefruit juice. If a Greyhound comes with a slice of lime, the Virgin Greyhound will too. To you it's a savings of about 135 calories as 1-1/2 ounces of gin is equal to 3 fat exchanges. Count the grapefruit juice in your diet – 1/2 cup contains 40 calories, 1 fruit exchange.

Virgin Mary is brunch perfect. A Bloody Mary without vodka. 6 oz. is only 35 calories. If you want lemon with your tomato juice ask for Virgin Mary with a twist of lemon. Virgin Mary can be ordered with or without salt on the edge of the glass. Another option – simply order Virgin Mary with the celery and you're sure to get the crunchy celery stock to stir your juice and chew on. It's better to chew on the celery than be tempted by cocktail peanuts!

Orange juice is the base for a Screwdriver. A Virgin Screwdriver is just plain o.j. Virgin Drivers usually are served on the rocks (over ice) without asking.

If a drink has a name it is somehow "socially acceptable," booze or not. No one notices that what you order is "different" if it has a bar name. Plain tomato juice is different – Virgin Mary is social. Try it, it's fun and another positive point – not only will you stay with your diet program – you'll know what a good time you've had! Cheers!

*Alcohol used in cooking evaporates when heated and does not need to be counted on your diet. The flavor remains (especially good with meats or mushrooms) but as the juices boil down the alcohol content disappears.

## DIET OUT OREGON . . .

### The Restaurants

**Clinkerdagger, Bickerstaff,**
**and Petts Public House**
**3775 S.W. Hall Blvd.**
**Beaverton, Oregon**

Hours: Lunch 11:30 am–2:00 pm Mon-Fri
5:30–11:00 pm Fri-Sat
Dinner 5:30–9:15 pm Sun-Thu
Reservations: Yes

Clinkerdagger, Bickerstaff and Petts, in English style, serves steaks, chicken, prime rib, seafood and house specials nightly.

Dinners come with a choice of steak soup or salad. All dinners also include steamed potatoes with buttery seasoning. The potatoes may be requested served without the butter. Baked potatoes are available ala carte.

Fresh steamed vegetables are ala carte and served with seasoned butter. The butter for vegetables may be held or served on the side. On special request, the kitchen will prepare a vegetable saute entree.

Steaks are char-broiled with the exception of steak Horatio. Approximate steak sizes are: small top sirloin 7-1/2 oz., large top sirloin 10-1/2 oz., and London broil 7 oz. Roast prime rib is approximately a 10-1/2 oz. cut.

All of the fish portions are 7 oz. to 8 oz. servings and the fish is baked or broiled. The salmon filet and market day fish (fresh changes daily) are favorites. Chicken dishes are sauteed.

A basket of fresh bread is served with all dinners. Butter is on the side and margarine is available on request.

Unsweetened fruit juice, diet Pepsi and artificial sweetener are available.

There are two dinner salads on the menu – Taco and Spinach.

Lunch features salads, special sandwiches, quiche and seafood. The fish is baked or broiled with the exception of the French fried shrimp.

Clinkerdagger, Bickerstaff and Petts tries to honor special diet requests.

The little "red" treat on dinner plates has a bit of sugar. It is strawberry ice and served to clean your palate so you may enjoy all the flavors of your entree!

**El Torito – Beaverton**
**12570 S.W. Center St.**
**Beaverton, Oregon 97005**

Hours: 11:00 am–11:00 pm Mon-Thurs
11:00 am-12:00 pm Fri-Sat-Sun
(Sunday Brunch 10:00 am-2:00 pm)
Reservations: Yes
Special Menus: Childrens

El Torito is a bright, modern Mexican style restaurant serving full meals, assorted ala carte specials and tasty Mexican salads. Tacos, enchiladas and tostadas come with your choice of beef or chicken and sauce can be ordered on the side. Chicken has been boiled. Combinations are served with rice and beans and your choice of lentil soup or green salad. Diet wise it is easier to order ala carte and specify what your preference is - thus only ordering what you need and will eat. Substitutions on full dinners are very limited.

Steaks are cooked on an open broiler and run 5 oz. – 8 oz. Broiled hamburgers (4 oz. patty) are on the lunch menu and may be requested at dinner. Condiments may be requested served on the side. Hamburgers are the only sandwich available.

Canned Mexican corn is the only hot vegetable available and is served without fat.

Diet R.C., unsweetened orange juice, coffee and tea are available and the full service bar will provide non-alcoholic beverages. Artificial sweetener is stocked.

The bar is lively, crowded and popular and will serve a Quesadilla appetizer (soft tortillas filled with melted cheese) without the guacamole and sour cream on request.

**Earthquake Ethel's Roadhouse**
**2970 S.W. Cedar Hills Blvd.**
**Beaverton, Oregon 97005**

Hours: Weekdays 11:00 am–2:00 am
Sat–Sun Noon to 2:00 am

Not all "Roadhouses" and dance halls are noted for their food and flexibility. Earthquake Ethel's is the exception! The music is soft at noon, the tables are filled and service is good. From 5:00 until 8:00 pm music is taped and after the 8:00 pm earthquake (unbelievable!) disco is the way of life! On Sunday children are welcome and family dining is noon–9:00 pm. Not only is the food good, the disco scene welcomes families and is diet legal — the choices are good.

Earthquake Ethel's offers a wide variety of broiled and roasted choices. The beef brochette (5–1/2 oz. lunch — 7 oz. dinner) chicken brochette (5–1/2 oz. lunch — 7 oz. dinner) broiled halibut (7 oz. lunch — 10 oz. dinner) roast turkey sandwich (3 oz.), roast beef sandwich (3 oz.), and coquille St. Jacques (7–8 oz. portion — dinner only) are examples. Serving sizes are as close as possible but do vary a bit by the cut.

Fresh vegetables, cooked without fat, are served with many entrees and are available ala carte. Steamed artichokes are a featured ala carte accompaniment.

Salads and rice pilaf are served with most lunch and dinner entrees. The oil and vinegar dressing is sugar free and the rice pilaf is cooked without oil as it is baked and steamed in the oven. One half cup serving of the rice equals only one bread exchange — 70 calories. If a salad meal is your choice, Shrimp and Crab Louie are available at both lunch and dinner.

Iced tea, grapefruit juice and tomato juice are available as well as coffee, tea and milk.

The crab stuffed tomatoes and fruit and cheese board are also popular with dieters.

Although Earthquake Ethel's is unable to tailor special menus, they are very willing to make substitutions to the extent that the substitutions can meet the dieter's requirements, says Paul Forchuk, Earthquake Ethel's president.

Special note: This restaurant is interested in persons on special diets and is in the process of adding other diet perfect items. Watch for them.

The full service bar will serve non-alcoholic beverages.

Grandma's Table
12255 S.W. Denney Road
Beaverton, Oregon 97005

Hours: Lunch 11:00 am–2:00 Mon-Fri
Dinner 4:00–10:00 pm Mon-Sat – 12:00–8:00 pm Sun
Sunday Brunch 9:00 am–12:00 pm
Reservations: Parties of 10 or larger
Special Menus: Children (Dinner and brunch)
Senior Citizen discount cards for dinners

Grandma's Table is a busy family style restaurant offering many entree choices that will easily (and quite economically) fit into a diet.

Dinner meals are served with a loaf of bread, kettle of chicken noodle soup, vegetables, potatoes and gravy. Help yourself. Meat entrees are served on diners individual plates, everything else is family style at the table. Chicken and dumplings are an order for two. They're a bowl and may have the gravy on the side – if requested.

Steaks (8 oz. – 9 oz. – 10 oz.) are broiled. Prime rib (10 oz.), pork chops, ham and turkey are roast or baked. Halibut and salmon are poached.

Oil and vinegar is the sugar free dressing at Grandma's and may be served on the side. Vegetables are canned varieties and cooked and served without fat.

Bread is served with a butter-margarine mix. Butter or margarine alone may be requested.

The low cal lunch is a broiled beef patty, cottage cheese with fruit, hard boiled egg, tomato and rye crisp.

Hamburgers are broiled 4 oz. patties. Condiments may be held or served on the side with burgers or any sandwich.

Grandma's snack is soup, salad and bread.

Tab, tea, coffee and milk are served and Sweet 'n Lo is on hand.

By helping yourself to accompaniments and ordering entrees cooked without added fats it is relatively easy to have foods in the amounts that best fit your needs. Doggie bags are available if your meat item is too large.

**Seahorse Bay Restaurant**
**10860 S.W. Beaverton/**
**Hillsdale Highway**
**Beaverton, Oregon 97005**

Hours: Mon-Th 11 am-9 pm – Fri-Sat 11 am-9:30 pm – Sun 1-9 pm
Reservations: Parties of 7 or more
Special Menus: Childrens – Senior Citizens

Seahorse Bay Restaurant is a dieters dream come true and one the entire family will enjoy! Everything cooked here is prepared over a wood fire without sauce or seasoning. The hot fire seals in moisture and brings out the true flavors of the food. At lunch fish portions are 6 oz. and dinner 9 oz. Some offerings include: ling cod, petrale sole, halibut, snapper and sturgeon. There is also scallops, catfish and a mixed seafood skewer. Poultry is not served but broiled steaks begin at 7 oz. and a 5-1/3 oz. broiled patty is available.

Dinners come with salad (or chowder) and there are three sugar free choices from which to choose. The 1000 Island is sugar free and has a mayonnaise base while the French and Italian are of an oil and vinegar origin.

Fresh and frozen vegetables are always available and are cooked without added fat. Vegies may be ordered ala carte but dinners (and most lunch plates) include a vegetable choice.

Butter and margarine are available and may be served on the side for the steamed potatoes and the rice is steamed without fat.

Diet beverages and artificial sweeteners are available and Seahorse Bay will try as hard as possible to meet patron needs.

If your meal only began to satisfy your cravings for fresh seafood, Seahorse Bay also has a Marketcase where you can purchase fish to take home.

**Pavillion Bar and Grill**
**10700 S.W. Allen Blvd.**
**Beaverton, Oregon 97005**

Hours: 7:00 am–10:00 pm
Reservations: Recommended

The Pavillion Bar and Grill "tries to please" says manager Chuck Hinman when referring to persons on special diets.

They allow substitution of fresh vegetables for potato, serve an oil and vinegar salad dressing that can be ordered on the side, stock fresh orange juice and have diet beverages and artificial sweetener.

Many of the meat entrees are broiled or sauteed and the breast of chicken has not been deep fried. Many seafood items also are not cooked in a deep fryer.

Butter is served (may be on the side for potato) and rice pilaf has been fried or cooked in oil.

The diet plates feature ground sirloin and fresh steamed vegetable platter.

The bar will serve non-alcoholic beverages on request.

*Special requests are honored with notice for banquets too.

*Overnight guests may also have special items requested via room service.

**Beef and Brew West**
**10555 S.W. Canyon Road**
**Beaverton, Oregon 97005**

**Beef and Brew East**
**17544 S.E. Stark**
**Portland, Oregon 97223**

Hours: 5:00–10:00 pm
Reservations: Yes
Special Menus: Childrens

Beef and Brew offers various grilled steaks, seafood choices and chicken. Dinners are complete with French bread, tossed salad and your choice of cottage fries or rice pilaf. The rice pilaf has been baked in a buttery broth.

The bread and salad are the first course and butter and salad dressings are on the side. The salad arrives family style for self serve and none of the dressings are sugar free. Oil and vinegar is available as are lemon slices if requested.

Grilled steaks can be ordered from 7 oz. – 12 oz. sizes (check with server for size of your cut choices), and the prime rib is roast. The broiled chicken breast is an 8 oz. serving and may be served without sauce or with the sauce on the side. Fish and seafood entrees are 6 oz. – 8 oz. portions. Cod and scallops are deep fried, scampi is sauteed in butter and lobster tails are broiled.

Baked potatoes are available ala carte with condiments always served on the side.

Beef and Brew tries to be flexible within limits of the menu and if your server is aware of your needs, they will try to be most helpful. Beef and Brew is easy to fit into your dietary needs as so much of the food comes plain to be dressed at the table.

Seating is in booths in an arena surrounding a large fireplace. Dinners can also be ordered to include beverages as an option. Diet beverages and artificial sweetener are available.

**Stuart Anderson's Cattle Company Restaurants**

**3800 SW Cedar Hills Blvd.**
**Beaverton, Oregon**

**425 E. Burnside**
**Gresham, Oregon**

**16323 SE McLoughlin Blvd.**
**Milwaukie, Oregon**

Hours: Mon–Thurs 11:00 am–10:30 pm
Fri–Sat 11:00 am–11:30 pm – Sun 11:00 am–10:00 pm
Reservations: Taken
Special Menus: Childrens

Stuart Anderson's, with its western theme and private individual dining booths, features char-broiled steaks, prime rib and Alaska king crab. The restaurant attempts to accomodate most dietary needs.

The house dinner salad (now a combination of lettuce, fresh mushrooms, cherry tomato, purple onion and croutons) may be topped with two sugar free dressing choices. The blue cheese has a mayonnaise base, vinegar and oil is seasoned. Salads are included with dinner as are ranch bread (French bread topped with buttery cheese, garlic and paprika) and your choice of baked potato, French fries or rice. The rice is steamed in chicken stock without fat and the potato topping (a whipped margarine base) will be served on the side if requested. Fresh vegetables are ala carte. The potato may be substituted for cottage cheese or sliced tomatoes. (Often the cottage cheese is served on a mini pineapple slice – check with waitress to see if your particular serving is on juice or syrup packed pineapple.)

Broiled steaks at dinner are London broil 9–10 oz., filet 7-1/2–8-1/2 oz., regular cut New York and top sirloin 9–10 oz. pre cooked weight. Roast prime rib is a 9–10 oz. serving.

Alaska king crab and lobster are served steamed or baked with drawn butter on the side. Crab is an 8–10 oz. serving. Lobster tails weigh 5–6 oz.

The lunch London broil serving is 6 oz. and prime rib is 7 oz. Noon time also features a taco salad that is a bed of greens topped with 6 oz. taco meat and vegetables. Toppings are served on the side for this specialty. The taco salad is served in a large flour tortilla that has been deep fried. There are also a variety of sandwiches at noon including French dip and broiled hamburgers.

Stuart Anderson's Restaurants do a pretty good job catering to special dietary requests and their advertisment claims "It'll make you feel good inside." *Travelers note: These are part of a chain and menu is standard.

**J's Family Restaurant**
**and Pie House**
**1715 S. Beavercreek Road**
**Oregon City, Oregon**

**J's Family Restaurant**
**and Pie House**
**At the Mt. Hood Exit I-205**
**15851 S.E. 82nd Dr.**
**Clackamas, Oregon**

Hours: 6:00 am–10:00 pm
Reservations: No

J's Restaurant and Pie House serves breakfast, soups, salads, sandwiches and full dinner meals with the whole family in mind. There are offerings for large appetites, small eaters and waist watchers.

Sandwiches include a choice of tossed salad (dressings have sour cream, mayonnaise or oil and vinegar bases), cup of soup, potato salad, or French fries. Butter, mayonnaise or any condiments may be omitted or served on the side. Good choices include ham, turkey, and French dip.

Hamburgers are fried. Patties are 3 oz. and 4 oz. servings before cooking. Burgers are served on a sesame seed bun and include tomatoes, lettuce, dressing and pickles. Condiments may be served on the side and mustard (a diet free condiment) is available on request.

Soups are home made and specials change daily. Piping hot vegetable is served daily. Soup may be ordered alone or with corn bread. (The corn bread comes with honey butter.) Plain butter or margarine is available on request.

Dinners may be ordered ala carte or as complete meals. Ala carte includes a choice of soup or salad, potato and bread and butter. Baked potatoes may be topped on the side. Vegetables may be substituted for potato. Vegetables are fresh, frozen and canned varieties without fat. A fresh vegetable plate may be requested.

Meat portions are approximately 4 oz. servings.

Waist watchers might enjoy the breast of chicken or top sirloin served with cottage cheese, fresh tomatoes and asparagus spears.

Salads are a good diet choice. Chefs salads with turkey, ham, Swiss and American cheese, egg, lettuce, and tomato are available in the regular portion or 1/2 size. Shrimp salads also have the 1/2 portion option.

J's always has fresh seasonal fruit and diet cola. Artificial sweetener is available.

J's are dependable restaurants to stop at along the road and will try to accomodate special requests within the range of their standard offerings. The menu is long, offers lots of food choices and the entire bill of fare is served from 11:30 until closing. During breakfast hours many items may be available on request.

*There are 23 home made pie specialties on the back of the menu – avoid temptation . . read only the inside selections!

| **Tebo's Restaurant** | **Tebo's Restaurants, Inc.** |
|---|---|
| **King City Plaza** | **19120 S.E. McLoughlin Blvd.** |
| **Tigard, Oregon** | **Gladstone, Oregon** |

Hours: 11:00 am-8:30 pm (Mon-Sat)
12:00–9:00 pm (Sun)
Special Menus: Kiddie Burgers, Dogs, Fish — (1/2 regular order & fries)

Every item at Tebós can be ordered ala carte. Foods are prepared fresh daily in their kitchens and pre-processed food items are not used.

Hamburgers have long been the house specialty and the 4 oz. burgers are char-broiled on order. It's cafeteria style so it's easy to talk directly to the cook for special requests on any item. Buns are toasted on the broiler without fat.

Sandwiches are all dressed at the condiment bar — self service. Turkey, ham, corned beef, roast beef, pastrami and Tillamook cheese are sandwich choices. Tenderloin steak sandwiches are broiled and served with a toasted bun.

The hamburger dinner steak is a broiled 8 oz. patty served with your choice of salad (there are 15), baked potato and beverage. Baked potatoes always have butter and sour cream on the side.

Soups are home made and change daily. Clam chowder is served on Friday. The chef salad is also a popular Friday special.

It is easy to have special requests met at Tebo's if you ask. The menu is simple and flexible.

Diet 7-Up, artificial sweetener and fresh fruit are always available.

* Warning: The desserts are home made and tempting . . . . especially the springtime strawberry shortcake! (If you ask they may have fresh sliced strawberries without the syrup.) Pies are the featured dessert year around.

**Sunnyside Inn**
**12605 S.E. 97th**
**Clackamas, Oregon**

Hours: 6:30 am–2:00 am
Reservations:

Sunnyside Inn is located off the 205 freeway near Clackamas Town Center and serves an ambitious menu for breakfast, lunch and dinner. Special buffets are added at lunch and dinner.

Salads may be ordered from the menu or you might choose the self service salad bar. Sunnyside Inn has a sugarless Italian salad dressing that has an oil-vinegar base.

All steaks are broiled and range from 6 oz. to 10 oz. cuts. The buffets generally offer roast beef. Chicken is available broiled or fried (in oil). Salmon is poached and filet of sole is sauteed.

Vegetables are frozen varieties that have fat added, are included with some entrees, and always available ala carte. Vegetables may be substituted for potato. Baked potatoes are always served with condiments on the side. Butter and margarine are both available.

Sandwiches are made to order and may have condiments held or served on the side. Hamburgers are broiled 5-1/3 oz. patties.

Diet beverages, artificial sweetener, fruit and unsweetened fruit juice are always served.

There is a diet plate at breakfast. Special requests are not encouraged. The buffets allow patrons to choose preferred items and many choices are ala carte.

The lounge will serve non-alcoholic beverages.

**High Rocks Pub**
**915 82nd Avenue**
**Gladstone, Oregon 97027**

Hours: 11 am–11 pm
Reservations: Large Groups Only

In a true sporting spirit High Rocks Pub offers something for just about any diet.

The minor league offers diet pop, iced tea, coffee, milk and fruit juice. And if you are with a group of major leaguers the bar will provide plain tomato juice, soda water with a twist of lemon or lime or a diet soda for your pleasure.

The infield specials include a salad bar that has a variety of lettuce, cauliflower, frozen peas, cucumber, onions, beets and carrots to mention a few of the choices for the do it yourself salad. Cole slaw, potato, macaroni and carrot raisin salad also make their appearance from time to time. There are two sugar free salad dressings – blue cheese with a mayonnaise base and the house dressing – a tangy oil and vinegar. The salad bar can be a meal in itself or it comes with your favorite sandwich. Sandwich condiments are all listed on the menu and may be held or served on the side. Some favorites include the "Three Strikes," a 3-1/2 oz. breast of turkey with 1-1/2 oz. of American Cheese, lettuce, tomato on sourdough bread, or "The Hole in One," ham (3-1/2 oz.) and Swiss (1-1/2 oz.) on rye bread. The "Knock Out" is a delicious warm corned beef (3-1/2 oz.), Swiss Cheese (1-1/2 oz.) combination with lettuce, tomato and mayo piled high on rye. The "One Hand Dunk" offering is a tasty French dip filled with 4 oz. of thin lean roast beef and a tasty au jus.

Complete dinners (salad bar, homemade soup, baked potato and a roll) include broiled entrees, an 8 oz. beef filet and 10 oz. chopped steak. Butter and sour cream for the potato are served on the side.

There is also a shrimp or crab salad (3 oz. seafood) on the menu.

Upon request any ingredient may be left off a sandwich and special reqeusts are cheerfully honored if at all possible.

High Rocks Pub is a great clean, casual place for the whole family and the same menu is served all hours.

**The Gazebo Gallery**
**Restaurant**
**11 Mt. Jefferson Terrace**
**(in Mountain Park)**
**Lake Oswego, Oregon 97034**

Hours: Lunch 11:45 am–3:00 pm Tue-Sun
Dinner 6:30–9:00 pm Thurs-Sat
Reservations: Yes

The Gazebo is a tranquil restaurant that mingles new artistry with fresh foods of the season. The restaurant is unique in structure and has an ever-changing menu that reflects the mood of the season.

The Gazebo serves fresh foods of the season — no preservatives or prepared ingredients — and is willing to share ingredients in a particular dish if asked. Nothing is deep fried. Seafood is poached, sauteed or baked and sauces served with entrees are made without sugar and may be served on the side.

Popular salads may be topped with a fresh sugar free dressing made with a tasty combination of oil, vinegar, lemon juice and herbs.

Seasonal vegetables are all fresh and included with entrees. Fresh fruits of the season are always available.

Butter is served and can be held or on the side of potatoes. Potatoes can also be substituted for extra vegetables. The home-cooked rice has been prepared with olive oil or butter.

Iced tea and mineral water are popular with dieters and artificial sweetener is not available.

Chef Palma skillfully prepares food served and when making reservations check on the current dishes being served. Much attention is given to special requests with items available and checking ahead will help you plan what will be right for you.

(*Warning — tempting desserts are also freshly baked.)

**Walrus and The Carpenter**
**15900 Boones Ferry Road**
**Lake Oswego, Oregon 97054**

Hours: 11:00 am–9:00 pm (Mon-Thu)
11:00 am–10:00 pm Fri-Sat)
Reservations: No
Special Menu: Children

The Walrus and The Carpenter is a casual family restaurant or a good place to relax with friends. Lunch and dinner features include fresh seafoods, sandwiches, soup, salad and burgers. After 5 special entrees are added.

The fresh fish change daily and may be cooked broiled or poached.

Burgers are 5 oz. grilled patties and any condiments may be held or omitted. There are eight combination burgers to choose from. All burgers are served with fresh fruit and your choice of soup (home made), salad or fries. Sandwiches are made to order and come with soup, green salad or potato salad. There are 14 combinations on the menu all with unique names and tasty fillings. Special sandwich requests are made from ingredients available.

Deep fried fish, scallops, oysters, shrimp and clam strips with shrimp salad and fries are available in three portion sizes.

At dinner scallops and scampi are sauteed in butter and wine. Alaska crab legs and clam are steamed. The 8 oz. top sirloin is usually grilled. Since broiling facilities are available request the steak broiled to cut down fats. Rice pilaf that is not cooked with oil is served.

Five entree salads are available and served with wheatberry bread. Butter and margarine are available.

Diet beverages, artificial sweetener, fresh fruit or unsweetened fruit juice are stocked.

Marc Hansen, owner of The Walrus and The Carpenter says to ask, the staff will try to honor all requests.

**Biffs Seafood Restaurant**
**12840 S.E. Stark**
**Portland, Oregon 97233**

Hours: 11:30 am–10:45 pm – Closed Sunday
Reservations: No
Special Menus: Childrens and Light Eaters

Biffs is a great place to "diet out." Seafood can be ordered practically any style, seafood salads are popular and a sugar free oil and vinegar dressing is available. Salads can be ordered in full or half portions.

Biffs will poach fish. Halibut is available in 5-6 oz. and 8-10 oz. portions. The fish of the day is always fresh and comes in 5-6 oz. or 8 oz. servings. Filet of sole may be ordered in two sizes – 5 oz. and 7 oz. Other seafood portions run 6 to 8 oz.

Canned vegetables and fresh tomatoes are available and vegetables come with many entrees or may be ordered ala carte. Substitution of vegetables for potato is also allowed. Fat has not been added to the vegetables and potato topping may be requested on the side. Butter and margarine are both available. Rice pilaf has been fried or cooked in oil.

Diet Rite and artificial sweetener are served. The bar will provide non-alcoholic beverages.

The light eaters portions are popular with dieters. Light meals come with soup or salad, vegetable or potato and a choice of fish and chips, grilled sole or a fresh filet of halibut. The light eaters choices may be ordered poached instead of grilled to save calories and fat exchanges.

"Biffs will honor special diet requests within reason," says owner Ronald Gustafson and "try to accomodate as many people as we can."

**Carnival**
**2805 S.W. Sam Jackson**
**Park Road**
**Portland, Oregon**

Hours: 11:00 am–9:00 pm Mon-Thurs – 11:00 am–10:00 pm Fri-Sat
Closed Sunday
Reservations: Not necessary
Special Menus: Childrens 1/6 lb Hamburger and Diet Plate

The candy striped hamburger and sandwich restaurant carved into the side of the hill is a hit with families and diet flexible as you dress your broiled burger from the condiment bar to your specifications!

Burgers come in three patty sizes (1/2 – 1/4 – 1/6 lb) and are broiled to order and served on warm buns.

Sandwich condiments may be held, served on the side or chosen from the "burger bar." The thinly sliced white breast of turkey sandwich has 3-1/2 oz. of turkey; corned beef and ham are a 4 oz. serving per sandwich and franks are 6 oz. Seafood is popular in the deviled crab or shrimp sandwiches.

Salads are the only available vegetables and the fresh mixed greens may be topped with a sugar free Italian dressing. The dressing may be served on the side and has an oil and vinegar base. Unsweetened fruit juice is not available.

The diet special consists of 1/4 lb broiled patty, tomato and cottage cheese salad, rye crisp and a drink. Tab, iced tea and coffee are dieters choices. Artificial sweetener is available and margarine is served.

The lively atmosphere and simple fare make the Carnival popular. You can eat indoors or in the summer enjoy your food outside at the picnic tables. Service is efficient and cafeteria style.

**The Crab Bowl**
**Restaurant and Market**
**7958 S.W. Barbur Blvd.**
**Portland, Oregon**

Hours: Sun 1:00–8:00 pm – Mon-Thu 11:00 am-9:00 pm
Fri-Sat 11:00 am–10:00 pm
Reservations: No
Special Menus: Junior and Senior

The Crab Bowl Restaurant and Market has an informal atmosphere and dungeness crab is a specialty. The crab salads are special with 8 oz. of crab. Whole crabs run 1-1/2–2 lbs and can be ordered whole, cracked, steamed and barbequed.

Fish and seafood choices are endless (nearly 80 items) and any item listed as deep fried on the menu may be ordered cooked in the steamers. Salads may be ordered with oil and vinegar on the side. House dressings are not sugar free.

Seafoods are available to take home, cooked from the restaurant or fresh and frozen from the Seafood Market.

French fries are the only potatoes served. Butter and garlic rolls are served on request. Seafood sandwiches are offered and the butter or mayonnaise may be held or will be served on the side.

Diet cola and sparkling water are available and the coffee, tea and iced tea are bottomless. Artificial sweetener is available.

Seafood – any type – fried or steamed is the house specialty and on seafood is where all effort is put forth and people wait in line – often outside – to consume. Portion sizes vary from item to item so check with server for serving size.

**Crepe Faire**
**133 S.W. 2nd & Pine**
**Portland, Oregon**

Hours: 7:30-10:00 pm – Closed Sunday
Reservations: Yes

Crepe Faire specializes in the preparation of crepes served with a variety of fillings and sauces. There are the traditional rolled crepe and a house feature is the mushroom spinach gateau, a tower of delicate flat crepes served in wedges. Seafood crepes and salads are also popular.

Salad dressings can be served on the side and Crepe Faire offers sugarless dressing based in oil and mayonnaise. Fresh, seasonal vegetables are available, some included with entrees, others ala carte. The vegetables are served without added fat. Butter is available. Potatoes are not served.

The popular seafood and poultry entrees are approximately 6 oz. portions.

Fresh fruit and unsweetened juice are available on request and diet beverages are served. Artificial sweetener is not available. The bar will serve non-alcoholic beverages, and the kitchen will try to honor special food requests of patrons.

## CHURCH'S CHICKEN

**50th & S.E. Powell**
**Portland, Oregon**

**188th & Stark**
**Portland, Oregon**

**5721 N.E. Union**
**Portland, Oregon**

**707 N.E. Weidler**
**Portland, Oregon**

**122nd & S.E. Powell**
**Portland, Oregon**

**1915 S. Willamette**
**Eugene, Oregon**

**1899 Olympic**
**Springfield, Oregon**

**2099 River Road**
**Eugene, Oregon**

**Also in Klamath Falls, Roseburg and Medford**

Church's features fried chicken from large scalded birds. Mr. Dodd Fisher, franchise operator, says the birds are processed with hot water prior to cooking to eliminate outer fat. Birds average 2.6 pounds and the average piece is 5.1 oz. Customers are given their choice of pieces when ordering. Chicken is fried in a vegetable base shortening.

White rolls are served with all chicken orders and a margarine patty is available on request. Corn can be ordered plain and diet Pepsi is served.

**Dan and Louis Oyster Bar**
**208 S.W. Ankeny**
**Portland, Oregon**

Hours: 11:00 am–Midnight Sun–Thurs
11:00 am–1:00 am Fri–Sat
Reservations: 5 or more

Dan and Louis Oyster Bar is a Portland institution. The restaurant was established in 1907 and decor is all nautical surroundings and historical bric a brac. Fresh Yaquina Bay oysters (the house specialty), Crab and Shrimp Louies are generous and patron favorites.

Crab and Shrimp Louies are available in three sizes – 3 oz. 6 oz. and 9 oz. of seafood with lettuce and dressing can be omitted or served on the side. Lemon wedges are available. A smaller amount of salad with shrimp is included on seafood plates.

Seafood cocktails, crab, shrimp, oyster are full 3 oz. portions and the sauce may be held.

Most seafood plates (scallops, shrimp, oyster, fish and chips and geoduck) are deep fried. The king crab steak can be steamed. Portions are 5 oz. to 8 oz. Warm rolls and butter are served with seafood. Smaller portions are available until 3:00 pm and after 10:00 pm.

The oyster stew is outstanding. It is rich and creamy with milk and butter and is available with regular or double oyster portions. Oyster, crab, shrimp and tasty combination stews are made to order. Butter on top can be omitted.

The Oyster Bar sticks to standards on the menu and will be adding tomatoes, and peaches with cottage cheese.

Diet Tab and artificial sweetener are served.

**Delevan's**
**1425 N.W. Glisan**
**Portland, Oregon**

Hours: Lunch 11:00 am–2:00 pm – Dinner 5:30 pm–10:00 pm
Sunday Brunch 1:00 am–2:00 pm
Reservations: Please

Delevan's Restaurant is a remodeled early 1900 firehouse. The upstairs is elegantly treated, candlelit with emphasis on customer service. Downstairs there is a bar that also serves light meals.

Delevan's has one of Portland's few real charcoal broilers using mesquite hardwood charcoal that is chemical free. Veal is the specialty of the house and all vegetables and fruits are fresh. Juice is even squeezed fresh on the premises.

Dinners may be ordered as full dinners or ala carte. The full dinners include soup and salad. The vinagerette dressing is sugar free and may be served on the side.

Beef filets (6-7 oz.) are charcoal broiled and poultry entrees (6-8 oz. portions) are sauteed or baked. There are several seafood choices (6-8 oz. portions) that are either sauteed, baked or charcoal grilled. Entrees are well out of the ordinary and generally served with fine sauces that can be served on the side.

Dinners may be ordered ala carte and light meals are also available. The owner suggests the vegetable frittata as a diet choice. It is a baked open-faced omelette filled with fresh vegetables. On the full dinner menu there is also a composed vegetable plate which is a changing assortment of stuffed, cooked and raw vegetables surrounding a vegetable vol au vent. Extra care is given each menu item!

Diet 7-Up and cola and Perrier water are available as is artificial sweetener.

Delevan's attempts to honor special requests at the table and will go the "extra step" to meet patrons' needs if possible. Special requests may be discussed at the time of reservation.

**'Enry Beazely's**
**Clackamas Town Center**
**(inside the shopping mall)**
**Clackamas, Oregon**

**Enry Beazely's**
**(Hollywood District)**
**2000 N.E. 40th Ave.**
**Portland, Oregon**

Hours: Hollywood District 11:00 am–10:00 pm daily
Town Center – Mall hours

'Enry Beazely's house specialty is an authentic order of English style fish and chips or deep fried seafood.

The menu has also included the dieter and offers a diet plate consisting of 6 oz. baked cod, cottage cheese, lettuce, tomato and rye crisp. Sauces (tarter and red) are served on the side.

There is a self-serve (1 helping) salad bar with a variety of fresh vegetables and generally cole slaw. The clam chowder is a thick creamy Boston style soup available in 8 oz. and 16 oz. portions. A pat of butter is floated in each serving and may be held on request.

Hamburgers and hot dogs are self dressed at the condiment bar. Patties and franks are 1/4 lb. before cooking (Hollywood district only)

Tab and iced tea are served. Artificial sweetener is available.

All items are available ala carte allowing some flexibility. 'Enrys are cheerful and clean and most accomodating within the limited range of the menu.

**Food In Bloom**
**8610 S.W. Terwilliger**
**Portland, Oregon**
**245-8083**

Hours: 10:00 am–7:00 pm Tues-Sat

Want something special for your next occasion or a gourmet treat for the family? Call caterers Jim Harris and Annie Stettner. The location is new but the duo is experienced and dedicated to serving fine foods.

Food In Bloom does not work within boundaries and the owners find a challenge in preparing and presenting foods to meet your special needs. If it's a low calorie gourmet offering you desire they will work with you for the perfect item or items. No occasion is too large or too small.

The deli case features many items not often served in this country. Many are rich but others may be worked in a diet. The sausage stuffed brioche (it's baked right in the rich bread), pithiviar, a free standing puff pastry French meat pie, and quiche (a specialty) are popular.

For the family celebration, wedding or your "diet club" picnic Food In Bloom will prepare and present carefully selected items for the occasion. Sugarless desserts are also available on request.

**Goldberg's**
**1329 Lloyd Center**
**Portland, Oregon**

Hours: 11:00 am–8:30 pm
Reservations: No

Goldberg's, a cafeteria style restaurant with a take-out deli counter, offers something for everyone as you work your way along the counter.

First come the desserts so dieters look ahead to the salads. Their roquefort dressing is made without sugar and has a mayonnaise base.

Most meats are roasted and hand carved to order. Meat portions generally are 3-1/2–4 oz. portions and can be served as part of a full meal or delicious sandwiches. Sandwiches are warm, made to order and may have the butter held. Mustard, sauerkraut and kosher dills are available to add to your sandwich choice and all are sugar free and low calorie, however, high in salt content. The Vienna style corned beef sandwich on fresh rye (3-1/2–4 oz.) has long been a favorite.

The steam tables offer a variety of entrees that might include cabbage rolls or short ribs with potatoes, vegetables, rolls and butter. Vegetables are cooked and served without added fat and may be fresh, frozen or canned. Vegetables are included on full meal items and are always available ala carte.

Soup is homemade daily and roast turkey is a Friday night special.

Diet beverages and artificial sweetener are available.

The Goldberg cafeteria line offers great flexibility for persons on special diets as you order what you like, watch it being "put together" and can have condiments held and will know just what you are eating because when you reach the end of the line your meal is "tailor made," a co-operative effort of Goldbergs and you!

**Hamburger Patti's**
**4239 N.E. Fremont**
**Portland, Oregon 97213**

Hours: Tues-Sat 11:00 am-9:00 pm
Reservations: Not Taken

Hamburger Patti's is best known for its juicy grilled burgers, but also offers a variety of well prepared sandwiches, diet plate choices, a chef's salad and other specialties. If special needs are made known, Hamburger Patti's waitresses and managers will go out of their way to see special needs are met if at all possible within their operation and food available.

Sugar free blue cheese dressing (has a buttermilk — mayonnaise base) and a tasty seasoned oil and vinegar combination may be served on the side to dress tossed green or chef salad choices. The chef salad is available in full or 1/2 portions.

The fresh roast beef sandwich has 4 oz. of meat and condiments may be requested on the side.

The diet plate is a grilled 1/4 lb meat patty and tossed salad and also available on request is a baked fish diet plate. The baked cod is a 4 oz. portion.

The burgers are grilled (regular are a 1/4 lb. patty) and are available in many varieties — regular — cheese — double — and "Big George" (everything plus — grilled onions, mushrooms and black olives). Tomato, lettuce, Neusihin pickles, and sliced onion come on all burgers between the halves of sesame seed buns. Mayonnaise and margarine may be requested on the side.

Diet Tab, hot and iced tea, apple juice, milk, coffee, V-8 and tomato juice are served and artificial sweetener is available.

Hamburger Patti's is a neighborhood restaurant that takes pride in its food and good care of its patrons.

**Henry Thiele's**
**2305 W. Burnside St.**
**Portland, Oregon**

Hours: 7:00 am–10:00 pm

"The Henry Thiele menu is large and practically all diets can be accommodated," says owner Margaret Thiele. Henry Thiele's menu changes daily and there is always a wide range of broiled and roasted entrees as well as salads and sandwiches. Many customers have been regular patrons for decades.

Meat, poultry and seafood entrees average 4-6 oz portions and any sauces or gravies may be held or served on the side. Potatoes with entrees may be topped on the side or vegetables substituted for the potato. Vegetables are seasonal and may be fresh, frozen or canned varieties. Many entrees have vegetables included but vegetables are also always available ala carte. Rice pilaf has not been fried or cooked in oil.

Hamburgers are 4 oz. broiled patties and may be dressed on the side.

Salad dressing may also be served on the side and the oil and vinegar is without sugar. Lemon slices are also available for salads.

Iced tea, coffee, carbonated water are served. Artificial sweetener, fresh fruit or unsweetened juice are always available.

Thiele's is proud of their long time reputation for good food and service and will co-operate on special requests within reason.

**Hilaires Encore**
**622 S.W. Washington**
**Portland, Oregon 97205**

Hours: 6:00 am–9:00 pm
Reservations: Recommended

Restauranteur Larry Hilaire has long been feeding Portlanders and meeting special needs with menu offerings.

There is a choice of meat items that have been roasted or broiled and the special diet meal is thin rare beef, cottage cheese and a hard roll. Non-fried seafood is offered in 4 oz. portions. Butter is served and margarine is available on request.

Salads can have dressings held and be topped with sugarless vinegar and oil. Fresh and/or frozen seasonal vegetables are served with entrees and cooked without fat. Vegetables may be substituted for potato.

Fresh fruit or unsweetened fruit juice is available and diet beverages and artificial sweetener are served.

**Horatios**
**4850 S.W. Macadam**
**Portland, Oregon**

Hours: Mon-Fri Lunch 11:30 am-2:00 pm — 11:45 am-2:30 pm Sat.
Reservations: Yes 5—
Special Menu: Childrens Sirloin & Teriyaki Steak Portions Available

Horatio's, with its nautical decor and waitress dressed like wenches and waiters in knickers, serves steaks, chicken, seafood, and house specials nightly. The menu offers good choice and may easily accomodate most diets.

There is a choice of clam chowder or tossed salad with dinner entrees for openers. All dinners also include your choice of a fresh lightly steamed vegetable (with hollandaise sauce that may be held or requested on the side) or a baked potato that may also be topped on the side if requested. Special vegetable dishes (5 are sauteed) are also available at dinner. Prime rib is roasted and steak grilled.

All of the fish is baked or broiled and portions are 7-8 oz. servings. The salmon filet and market day (fresh changes daily) are favorites.

Chicken Wellington (5 oz.) and Chicken Florentine (5 oz.) may have the hollandaise on the side.

A basket of fresh dark rye bread is served with all dinners. Butter is in little individual serving dishes and margarine is available on request.

Unsweetened fruit juice, diet Pepsi and artificial sweetener are available.

There are two dinner salads — Taco and Spinach — also on the menu.

Lunch features salads, special sandwiches, quiche and seafood. Hamburgers are broiled (8 oz. patty) and the fish is generally baked or broiled with the exception of the french fried shrimp.

Horatios tries to honor special diet requests and offers a flexible menu and choices are standard for everyone so much substitution is unnecessary.

The large windows and terraced floors give most diners a view of the mighty Willamette River.

**Jake's Restaurant**
**401 S.W. 12th**
**Portland, Oregon**

Hours: Lunch Mon-Fri 11:30 am–3:00 pm
Dinner Mon-Thurs 5:00–11:00 pm – Fri-Sat 8:00–12:00 pm
Sun 5:00–10:00 pm

Jake's Famous Crawfish Restaurant has become a Portland institution specializing in seafood since 1892. Emphasis is on the seafood featuring fresh salmon, halibut, oysters and a wide variety of foods prepared broiled, poached, baked or sauteed. Halibut, salmon and most entrees are 8-10 oz. portions. Fresh baked oysters can be ordered with Italian seasonings in a spicy tomato, bacon and cheese pepper pan, as Rockefeller or on a combination oyster plate. Real oyster lovers order them on the half shell. The Rockefeller as well as other dishes may be served without excessive or any oils at all.

Hot fresh vegetables come with entrees and generally are seasoned and buttered, however, upon request, vegetables may be simply steamed and served without seasonings. The accompanying rice pilaf is not cooked in oil or fried. Baked potatoes are served with steaks or available ala carte and topping may be requested on the side. If you order a steak or steak-seafood combo and prefer additional vegetables, they may be substituted for the rice or potato.

Steaks are broiled and include top sirloin in 10-12 oz. cuts and 7-9 oz. filet mignon.

Although Jake's does not feature a diet plate they allow substitutions on practically everything on the menu and with the variety of seafood and the varied cooking equipment, they can cook their food to just about any person's liking and need. Broiled halibut, salmon, scampi, petrale sole, scallops, perch and red snapper seem to be favored by dieters as they are low fat meats with only 55 calories to the ounce.

Crusty French bread and butter are served with entrees and margarine is available.

Salads may be topped with a sugarless oil-vinegar and a popular noon time item is the Crab Louie that may have the dressing served on the side or be served with cocktail sauce and fresh lemon wedges.

The fresh crawfish are served when in season and come in shells for a do it yourself treat!

The full service bar will serve non-alcoholic beverages to add to your over all enjoyment and "diet-out" perfect meal.

P.S. If your serving is too large, ask for a doggie bag and have left over lunch the next day!

**John's Meatmarket**
**115 N.W. 22nd**
**Portland, Oregon**

Hours: Lunch 11:30 am–2:30 pm (Mon-Fri)
Dinner 5:00–11:00 pm (Mon-Thu)
5:00–12:00 pm (Fri-Sun)
Reservations: Yes
Special Feature: Suppertime Split

John's Meatmarket offers a wide variety of lunch and dinner items in a spacious warm atmosphere. Menu specialties include diet perfect broiled steaks, poached salmon, oven poached halibut and tempting salads.

Steaks are broiled top sirloin (12 oz. and 8 oz.), New York (12 oz.), filet mignon (6 oz., 8 oz., 12 oz.) and a chopped sirloin (12 oz.), that comes covered with mushroom sauce that can be held or served on the side. All dinners include your choice of soup, garden salad or spinach salad, vegetables and pan fried rice or French fries. Baked potatoes are available ala carte and may have topping on the side.

Columbia River salmon is an 8 oz. filet. It can be broiled (request lemon butter on side, if desired) or poached in a white wine with lemon, onion, green pepper and seasonings. The 8 oz. halibut filet is poached in butter and white wine.

John's Meatmarket offers a super option for persons on modified diets or lighter eaters, the **suppertime split.** Two people in the same party order the same entree from the regular menu (specialties, fish or steak), ask for the suppertime split, and they each receive one-half portion of the entree plus an individual choice/serving of soup or garden salad. Together you pay for just one meal. The suppertime split is a standard menu feature! This takes care of the temptation to "eat just a bit more," solves the doggie bag problem if you're not going straight home, and is very economical!

Sandwich choices are offered at dinner as are dinner salads.

Lunch offers a variety of sandwiches, house specialties, and has a unique light lunch section that features your choice of a large salad or soup and small salad or soup and 1/2 sandwich. Oil and vinegar is the only sugar free dressing. Soups are home made and include a choice of a thick rich vegetable steak soup, cold gazpacho, and ever changing soup of the day. Salad choices are spinach, shrimp and zucchini, chicken and chefs. Half sandwich choices are crabby-beef (thin slices of beef on a toasted English muffin, topped with crab, asparagus and Bernaise sauce) and crab and cheese (dungeness crab on a toasted English muffin with cheddar cheese sauce).

Hamburgers are large 8 oz. (before cooking) patties of sirloin served on toasted sourdough or buns with a variety of condiments.

Lunches that are served with French fries may have cottage cheese substituted for the fries on request.

The taco salad is popular at both lunch and dinner and is a large salad featuring seasoned ground beef, cheddar cheese, olives, tomatoes on a lettuce bed with tortilla chips and salsa.

Diet pop is available and the bar will serve non-alcoholic beverages. Food is also served in the lounge.

John's Meatmarket is flexible and does a very good job of honoring patron requests and meeting special needs.

**L'Auberge**
**2180 W. Burnside**
**Portland, Oregon**

Hours: Tues-Sat 6:00 pm-10:00 pm
Reservations: Yes (223-3302)

L'Auberge is a small intimate (11 tables — 35 person) restaurant with excellent service and a verbal menu. They offer a choice of 4-5 entrees daily which are served as part of a complete meal.

None of the dishes at L'Auberge are deep fried, cooked in heavy oils and sauces do not have added sugar. Most entrees have a sauce that can be served on the side. Roast or broiled meat entrees run 6-8 oz., poultry servings 8 oz. and fish and seafood is generally 8 oz. portions.

Vegetables are included with the entree and are fresh without added fat. When rice is served it is not cooked in oil.

The special house salad dressing is sugar free and has a condensed milk, oil, vinegar and spice base.

Artificial sweeteners and diet pop are not available but iced tea and soda water is served.

L'Auberge tries to honor requests made in advance to their small kitchen when doing so will not upset the general service and owner W. J. McLaughlin says "Weekdays are, of course, better for dealing with special diets!"

La Casa de Rios
4343 S.E. Hawthorne
Portland, Oregon 97215

Hours: 6:30–11:00 pm Mon–Fri – 8:00–11:00 pm Sat–Sun
Reservations: No
Special Menu: Vegetarian

La Casa de Rios is a small neighborhood restaurant where people line up evenings and weekends for the home cooked Mexican specials.

Full meals and ala carte side orders are available and any sauces may be omitted or served on the side.

The special house salad dressing is sugar free and is a tangy combination of wine vinegar, soy oil, sesame spices, egg and fresh onion.

Soybean oil is the only fat used in preparation of Mexican dishes. The Spanish rice is even fried in the soybean oil as are meatless dishes.

The chicken enchilada is a large serving of cooked chicken mixed with sauce in a fresh tortilla. The large tostada comes with all the usual meat, vegetables and cheese with sauce on the side. Try the sugar free house dressing on it. Seafood soup is a Friday special.

Diet R.C., mineral water, soft drinks and assorted beers are served along with coffee, tea and milk. Artificial sweetener is not available.

La Casa de Rios is family owned and operated and ordering ala carte is the best way to adapt your diet to their menu as many items are starchy.

**Lakeside Gardens**
**16223 S.E. Foster Road**
**Portland, Oregon**

Hours: 5:00 pm–10:00 pm Tues-Thurs
5:00–11:00 pm Fri-Sat
4:00–9:00 pm Sunday

Lakeside Gardens was one of my first "diabetic" dieting out experiences. It was so positive I have enjoyed the ease and leisurely dining at this restaurant on many occasions. The lakeside setting is restful and beautiful year around.

Dinners are complete and include soup, salad, vegetable, potato, entree and rolls.

The soup is served in a tureen at the table. The soups vary daily with the season and I judge my portion by the variety. There is a sugar free salad dressing (Dieters Gourmet) available on request. This dressing is purchased in a health food store and has an oil and vinegar base.

The butter for rolls and potato is always served on the side. Margarine is available on request. If one bread is all you are allowed simply eat the potato (or rice which has been cooked with a small amount of margarine) and save the roll to feed to the ever hungry ducks waiting outside!

All meat entrees may be roasted to order and generally are 6 oz. to 10 oz. portions. 4 oz. portions are available on request. Chicken breasts and roast duck are 4 oz. to 6 oz. servings. Baked salmon and grilled halibut are available in 4 oz. to 6 oz. portions. The halibut has an egg type batter coating.

Vegetables are seasonal and may be fresh, frozen or canned and all are cooked and served without added fat. Extra vegetables may also be substituted for potato or ordered ala carte.

Diet beverages, artificial sweetener and fresh fruit or unsweetened fruit juice are always available and the full serve bar will serve non-alcoholic beverages.

The Lakeside Gardens will honor special food diet requests of their patrons and owner Virginia Abbott says, "we will alter all dinners for diets."

Special Note: Individual attention is given to a person with special dietary needs even in large group and banquet settings if needs are made known at time of reservation.

**London Grill**
**S.W. Broadway at Oak**
**in the Benson Hotel**
**Portland, Oregon**

Hours: 6:30 am–11:00 pm
Reservations: Requested at Dinner

The London Grill is a tasteful Old English setting in the historic Benson Hotel and service and food are high quality.

There are various broiled and roasted meat entrees (some nice veal dishes) and poultry and chicken entrees that have not been deep fried. Many house specials are prepared at your table.

Fresh seasonal vegetables come with entrees and you may request no butter or fat be added. Fresh fruit or unsweetened fruit juice is available. The only sugar free salad dressing is oil and vinegar.

Baked potatoes can be topped on the side or substituted for vegetables and the rice pilaf is baked. Butter is generally served and margarine is available on request.

The London Grill is able to handle most special requests for handling of menu items and will serve sauces on the side or omit them on request.

Diet beverages and artificial sweetener is available and the full service bar will provide non-alcoholic beverages.

**The Matterhorn**
**3 N.E. 82nd Ave.**
**Portland, Oregon**

Hours: 11:30 am–11:00 pm
Reservations: Lunch Parties of 5 or more – Dinner: Yes
Special Menus: Childrens – Vegetarian Selections

The Matterhorn is a Swiss family restaurant complete with cowbells, cuckoo clocks and waitresses in costumes. Swiss and American items are served.

All dinners are preceded by Swiss cheese fondue served with crusty bread. This is a tasty way to eat a bread exchange as vegetables may be substituted for potato.

The regular menu offers dishes that are prepared by broiling or roasting. Poultry portions are approximatey 5 oz. servings. Fish and seafood portions run 5 oz. to 7 oz.

Tossed green salad or home made soup comes with dinner entrees. Oil and vinegar is the only sugar free dressing and may be substituted for house dressings. Dressing can be requested on the side. Dinner salad entrees served include a fruit salad platter, Crab and Shrimp Louies.

Vegetables are served with entrees and are either fresh or frozen varieties. They are cooked and served without added fat. Rice pilaf has been cooked in oil and butter. Potatoes may be topped on the side. Butter is served with baskets of crusty bread. Margarine is available on request. Coffee, tea or milk come as part of the complete dinner.

At lunch the Matterhorn has a wide selection of hot specialty entrees, salads, sandwiches and diet choices. Sandwiches are made to order and may have condiments held or served on the side. Hamburgers are grilled 5 oz. patties. An interesting change from the sandwich-salad lunch is the cheese fondue assorted salad combination.

Diet plate choices include ground beef with cottage cheese and fruit, sliced roast beef with broiled tomato, broccoli and cabbage or a grilled halibut steak with broccoli and seasonal fresh fruit.

Diet cola, mineral water, artificial sweetener and fresh fruit are always available.

The Matterhorn staff will honor special requests depending on availability.

The full service bar will serve non-alcoholic beverages.

**McCormick and Schmick's**
**Oak Street Restaurant**
**235 S.W. First**
**Portland, Oregon**

Hours: Lunch 11:30 am–2:30 pm – Dinner 5:00–11:00 pm
Reservations: Advised

McCormick and Schmick's Oak Street Restaurant draws a lively cocktail crowd and the dining area is separated from the busy bar. Specials of the house include prime rib (10 oz. and 13 oz. cuts) and a unique alder-smoked salmon or fresh Oregon trout.

Salads are included with the entrees and your choice includes tossed green (vinegar and oil dressing is sugar free) or spinach salad. Fresh steamed vegetables accompany all dinner entrees as does fettucini. Extra vegetables may be substituted for the pasta. Crusty French bread and butter comes with entrees and margarine is available on request.

The average meat, poultry and seafood portion is a 7-8 oz. serving. The live Maine lobsters (they swim in a tank in the entry way) run about 1-1/2 pounds each. Halibut and salmon are available baked or broiled and the menu features many interesting sauteed seafood and veal dishes. Special sauces can be omitted or served on the side.

Fresh fruit or unsweetened fruit juice can always be ordered and diet beverages and artificial sweetener are on hand. Mineral water is also served.

McCormick and Schmick's is usually very receptive and adaptable to customers' special needs and requests for preparation of menu items. Seafood is fresh except when not in season and the board in the entry lists fresh items.

**Nendels**
**9900 S.W. Canyon**
**Portland, Oregon 97228**

Hours: Breakfast 7:00am-10:30 am – Lunch 10:30 am–2:00 pm
Dinner 5:00 pm–11:00 pm
Reservations: Yes
Special Menus: Childrens and Senior Citizens

Nendels is decorated colonial style with a firelit dining room and serves a wide variety of foods all day and the chef will adhere to any salt or fat diet request – if at all possible.

Breakfast can be ordered ala carte or from a variety of entrees. The ala carte offers a wide enough variety – can be cooked as you like – to accomodate even the strictest diet.

Lunch offers salads, sandwiches, hot and cold, that may have all condiments on the side as well as special luncheon entrees. The entrees and hot sandwiches come with your choice of soup or salad. The only sugar free salad dressing is oil and vinegar. A low calorie lunch with roast beef, soup, cottage cheese and fruit is featured daily.

A long time favorite of regulars at dinner has been the Columbia River Salmon served poached or broiled. Many broiled steaks are offered, roast prime rib, and the special Nendel chicken liver saute with onions and mushrooms are popular.

There are five dinner salads. Nendels pineapple boat is served with chicken salad garnished with fresh fruit and vegetables.

Full dinners include your choice of liver pate or tomato juice, soup or salad, rolls, vegetable and baked potato or rice pilaf. Butter is served and may be served on the side. The rice pilaf has not been fried or cooked in oil. Vegetables are either fresh or frozen and do have fat added.

Fresh fruit or unsweetened juice is available as are diet beverages and artificial sweetener.

Lighter portions are offered for junior and senior citizens at dinner and the bar will serve non-alcoholic beverages if ordered.

**Old Country Kitchen**
**10519 S.E. Stark**
**Portland, Oregon 97216**

Hours: 4:00 pm–12:00 am
Reservations: No (large banquets only)
Special Menus: Children – Senior Citizen

The Old Country Kitchen features seafood, chicken and is the home of the 72 oz. steak! Steaks are the house specialty and are ordered by size beginning with a 6 oz. tenderloin and graduating to the 72 oz. top sirloin steak (roast?).

The Saylor family has long had a reputation for good food and honoring patrons' requests on their menu items and there is some flexibility on the complete dinners to fit most dieter needs. Dinners include tomato juice, fresh relishes, salad (your choice of tossed or cole slaw), your meat entree, baked or French fried potatoes, a basket of warm French bread (plain and garlic butter are served on the side), your beverage and a scoop of ice cream. The dinner is high quality and a moderate price.

Salad dressings may be ordered on the side and house dressings are not sugar free, however, oil and vinegar and fresh lemon slices are available. If you choose to eat your starch allowance in the garlic bread simply substitute the potato for a vegetable. Vegetables are of a canned variety and do not have added fat. Potato topping is always served on the side and the special house sour cream, chive mixture is 45 calories per 1-1/2 tablespoon.

Steaks are grilled but may be cooked otherwise on request and usually come topped with a butter pat that will be held if you ask. Chicken (1/2 chicken is 16 oz.) can be baked in the convection oven if requested. Halibut steaks (8 oz. – 12 oz. and 16 oz.) can also be ordered baked in the convection oven. Lobster is also a featured item. Lemon and tarter sauce are always on the side as well as a choice of steak sauces.

Diet R.C. Cola is available, iced tea, coffee and milk. The full service bar will provide plain tomato juice, soda with a lemon or lime twist as well as the diet pop.

Hamburgers and steak sandwiches are the only sandwiches served and the ground meat is a very low fat mixture that is fried. The patty size is 6 oz.

Ice cream is the only dessert available and it comes with dinner. There is a choice of flavors (160 calories per 1/2 cup – 1 bread and 2 fat exchanges) and sherbet (120 calories per 1/2 cup – 1 bread and 1 fat exchange).

Go early – this popular restaurant generally has a wait! It should also be noted that these guidelines also follow banquet settings – where each person may order his choice off the menu if prearranged.

**The Old Spaghetti Factory**
**SW 2nd and Pine**
**Portland, Oregon**

Hours: 5:00–10:00 pm
Reservations: No
Special Menus: Children

The Old Spaghetti Factory serves a limited menu but there are items available that can be worked in on a special diet. The building recently was declared a historical landmark and there are authentic antiques throughout.

Salad comes with full dinners or a crisp salad bowl may be ordered with sourdough bread. The house oil and vinegar is sugarless. The garlic butter for the bread is served on the side.

Spaghetti is available with a variety of sauces or may be ordered with meatballs, sausage or slices of tenderloin.

The Spaghetti Factory is flexible within their limited menu.

1/2 cup of cooked pasta equals 70 calories — 1 bread exchange. I find it easiest to order the salad bowl with sourdough and a side of meatballs.

Diet pop and artificial sweetener are available.

**Prime Rib**
**5474 N.E. Sandy Blvd.**
**Portland, Oregon**

Hours: Open for Lunch 11:30 am – Open for Dinner 5:00 pm
Reservations: Yes
Special Menus: Childrens

Specialty of the house is the "King of Roasts" – Prime Rib. Also featured are a variety of steak and seafood items.

Prime rib dinners are available in three sized cuts, beginning with the 7 oz. petite cut. All prime rib dinners include soup or tossed salad, baked potato, Yorkshire pudding, and creamed spinach.

The home made house salad dressing has a mayonnaise base without added sugar. Vegetables can be substituted for potato and topped on the side if requested. Butter is served.

Steaks are broiled (top sirloin and filet mignon) and run 8 oz. to 10 oz. These are served with soup or salad and baked potato. Halibut is normally sauteed in butter and wine but can be broiled on request. The Mariners salad entree is fresh greens topped with salad shrimp, crab, asparagus and tomatoes. Your choice of dressing can be served on the side.

The lunch menu includes the prime rib, served as the Prime Liner (5-6 oz.). It comes with soup or salad, vegetables, French fries and a hot roll. The halibut is approximately 6 oz. at lunch. Various omelettes, sandwiches and salads are also available at noon.

The Prime Rib does not have a diet beverage but does serve iced tea. The bar will serve non-alcoholic beverages.

**Quinn's Mill**
**5310 S.W. Macadam Ave.**
**Portland, Oregon 97201**

Hours: 11:15 am–11:00 pm
Reservations: Yes

Nestled quietly along the Willamette, Quinn's Mill was one of the first restaurants to open in the John's Landing area. Quinn's Mill serves lunch and dinner and offers a champagne brunch on Sunday. The menu offers many items for a dieter's enjoyment.

The self serve salad bar is fresh, cold and crisp and offers a variety of vegetables and a sugarless oil and vinegar dressing. It's help your self to all the salad you can eat – no charge for return trips.

Steaks are broiled and roast prime rib is served. Meat portions average 10 oz. servings. Poultry is available (and served not deep fried) and is a 12 oz. serving. Sauces may be held or served on the side on request. If seafood is your choice, portions average 10 oz.

Fresh vegetables are available ala carte and have been prepared without added fat. Vegetables may be substituted for potato. The rice pilaf has not been fried or cooked in oil.

Diet beverages, fresh fruit or unsweetened juice are served and artificial sweetener is available.

The popular French onion soup is made from tasty chicken and beef broth combined with fresh onions that have been sauteed with about 1/2 oz. butter per serving. It is topped with French bread and 2 oz. bubbly Swiss cheese and at lunch can be a meal in itself or is a good combination with the salad bar. The soup is served hot and is homemade.

Sandwiches are popular noon fare and are made to order so butter, mayonnaise or any condiments may be held or served on the side. Hamburgers are thick broiled 6 oz. patties and are available with or without cheese.

Quinn's Mill offers specials daily that are often broiled meats or fresh fish items and they will make every effort to honor special food/diet requests.

The full service bar will serve non-alcoholic beverages.

**The Rafters**
**220 S.E. Spokane**
**Portland, Oregon**

Hours: Lunch Mon-Fri 11:30 am–2:00 pm
Fri-Sat 5:30 pm-11:00 pm
Dinner Mon-Thu 5:30 pm–11:00 pm
Reservations: Yes
Special Menus: Childrens

The Rafters Restaurant is housed in a refurbished warehouse with wooden rafters, an indoor garden and is spread out over several levels. House specialties include prime rib, steak and seafood.

Prime rib is roasted without seasonings and all other beef is broiled. Portion sizes are 8 oz. through 16 oz. There is a broiled marinated 6 oz. chicken breast and seafood includes steamed crab and lobster, scallops baked with butter and wine (which may be omitted) and snapper and salmon baked with butter, wine and seasonings. The butter/wine may be omitted.

Substitutions are not allowed and there is not a sugar-free salad dressing.

Fresh and frozen vegetables are available, some included with entrees, others ala carte.

Unsweetened fruit juice is available as are diet Pepsi and artificial sweetener.

Butter is served and may be ordered on the side for baked potatoes. The rice pilaf has been cooked in oil.

The Rafters will try to fill special requests within their limitations and welcomes a phone call in advance to be sure of their ability to meet a special need.

**Rosés Restaurant East**
**12329 N.E. Glisan**
**Portland, Oregon 97230**

**Rosés Restaurant**
**315 N.W. 23rd Avenue**
**Portland, Oregon 97210**

Hours: 7:00 am–11:30 pm Sun–Thurs
7:00 am–12:30 am Fri–Sat
Reservations: Large Groups

Rosés is a bustling informal restaurant known best for their dazzling desserts. The house has other specialties including lox and bagels, kosher sandwiches and home made chicken matzoh ball soup. The dinner menu not only includes a wide variety of sandwiches but full meals as well.

Oil and vinegar is the only sugar free salad dressing. The roast sirloin and breast of chicken, with sauce on the side fit into modified diets. There is a dinner special steak (10 oz.) top sirloin that is grilled, comes with salad, a bagel with butter on the side, vegetables and baked potato or rice. Substitutions are not allowed but by adding your own potato topping you can control the portions fairly easily. The rice has been cooked in oil or fried. The vegetables may be fresh, frozen or canned depending on the season.

Diet RC and artificial sweetener are available.

If a sandwich is your choice butter and or mayonnaise may be held or served on the side.

The smallest hamburger is a 4 oz. grilled patty.

The full service bar will serve non-alcoholic beverages.

**Silver Garden**
**210 S.E. Ash**
**Portland, Oregon**

Hours: Lunch M-F: 11:30 am – Dinner 5:30 pm – 10:30 pm
Reservations: Recommended

Nestled quietly "down by the tracks" is the Silver Garden Restaurant appropriately placed, as the dining room is actually a "retired" train diner.

Food is creatively served and the Silver Garden gives special attention to patrons with dietary requests.

There is always an abundance of fresh vegetables available which are normally sauteed in butter. On request the butter can be omitted. There are two sugar free salad dressings served regularly. The "house" is a tasty oil and vinegar base and the roquefort is made with sour cream.

Steaks are broiled to order and the menu offers a 10 oz. top sirloin, a tasty 5 oz. steak with giant shrimp (shrimp can be grilled or sauteed) for starters. The roast prime rib is a 10 oz. or 12 oz. serving and there is a lovely baked (8 oz.) chicken breast that is filled with (1 oz.) of cheese and can have the sauce served on the side. Baked shrimp (5 oz.) can also be worked in on the diet.

The house rice has about 85 calories per half cup (1 bread exchange 1/3 fat exchange) and is a tasty change from potato. But if potato is your choice topping can be served on the side if requested. Butter is the house standard but margarine is available upon request.

Diet beverages include a sugar free pop, iced tea and coffee. From the bar one may have plain tomato juice, orange or grapefruit juice.

For a relaxed evening or special occasion celebration Silver Garden has a unique setting, creative menu and willingness to fulfill special patron requests.

**Stanich's**
**Ten-Till-One**
**4915 N.E. Fremont**
**Portland, Oregon**

Hours: 11:00 am–1:00 am Mon–Sat
Reservations: Yes

Stanich's Ten-Till-One Tavern is home of the "World's Greatest Hamburger." The title was bestowed on the burger by Jack Pement of the Oregon Journal and judging by its following, he is right. Stanich's serves about 400 burgers a day.

A diet special – not exactly, the Ten-Till-One special includes a 4 oz. grilled beef patty, slice of ham (Canadian bacon style), a fried egg, bacon (2 half slices), a slice of cheese, tomatoes, lettuce, pickles, onion, special mayo and relish between the halves of a sesame seed bun. Regular hamburgers (4 oz. grilled patties) are served without the cheese, ham, egg and bacon. Condiments may be held and burgers are served with potato chips.

Beverages include a beer/wine and soft drink selection and sugar free Tab and Fresca are available as are coffee and tomato juice.

Stanich's uses the special burger ingredients to create other sandwich offerings (fried egg, ham, ham and egg and bacon and tomato to name a few). Tuna is also available.

The grill hours are 11:00 am–11:30 pm and food may be ordered to go.

**The Steamers**
**8303 N.E. Sandy Blvd.**
**Portland, Oregon**

Hours: 6:00 am–3:00 pm – 5:00–9:00 pm
Sunday Brunch 9:30 am–3:00 pm
Reservations: Yes
Special Menus: Childrens

At The Steamers the decor is as varied as the menu. Semi-private booths and tables, each decorated in its own fashion set the pace for meals with many choices that are diet legal.

Breakfast is a variety of the "standard" morning fare. On the side items may be ordered prepared your choice (like eggs poached or boiled), an order of plain toast, fresh melon and the like in amounts you need thus avoiding the extra "goodies" that come on combinations. (This saves your diet and your pocket book.)

Lunch and dinner both feature self serve salad bars and menu items. At noon the salad bar also includes a buffet option. The salad bar is complete with many fresh vegetables, a variety of home made salads and unique garnishes.

The Thousand Island salad dressing is sugar free and has a mayonnaise base. Dinners include the salad bar. At noon a luncheon salad is served with many menu choices and dressing is available on the side.

Dinners also include crusty French bread, your choice of baked potato, zesty rice, steak fries or gently cooked fresh vegetable. If potato or rice is your choice, vegetables are available ala carte. The rice has been cooked in butter. Potato topping (a 60-40 butter-margarine blend) is available on the side. Plain butter or margarine is available on request.

Steaks are broiled and the New York is a hearty 10 oz. cut. Top sirloin is available in 8 oz. and 10 oz. portions. If roast beef is your choice – try the prime rib. Chicken portions run about 8 oz. at dinner and salmon and halibut are 7 oz. Sauces may be held or requested on the side.

Special menu features are the crock of butter clams served with lemon and drawn butter and the Steamer's Seafood Catch – a combination of shell fish in a crock of seafood nectar.

Hamburgers are broiled 6 oz. patties and condiments can be served on the side.

Diet beverages, fresh fruit, unsweetened fruit juice and artificial sweetener are available.

The Steamer's menu is flexible and the kitchen staff tries to honor special requests and needs

**Thunderbird/Red Lion**
**Jantzen Beach**
**Hayden Island Drive**
**Portland, Oregon**

**Thunderbird/Red Lion**
**Lloyd Center**
**Portland, Oregon**

**Thunderbird/Red Lion**
**Portland Center**
**310 S.W. Lincoln**
**Portland, Oregon**

**Thunderbird**
**Coliseum**
**1225 N. Thunderbird Way**
**Portland, Oregon**

Reservations: Suggested
Special Menus: Children

The Thunderbird/Red Lion kitchens feature quality ingredients and flexible menus. Coffee shops and dining rooms are well stocked and make a real effort to honor special requests.

Breakfasts come in a wide range of combination plates and ala carte items. Ala carte items are easily prepared to meet special requests. Fresh fruit is always available.

Lunch and dinner menus feature offerings in a wide range in both coffee shop and dining rooms. Food is the same high quality in both kitchens with dining room service being more formal.

Soups are home-made. Sandwiches may have condiments omitted or served on the side. French fries can be substituted for cottage cheese or often a cup of soup.

Blue cheese dressing is home-made without added sugar and has a mayonnasie base. Vinegar and oil is also available without sugar. Lunch menus feature nice salad choices and salad (entree type) may be requested at dinner even if not on the menu. The seafood Louies have approximately 4 oz. shrimp or crab. Dinner salads are tasty combinations of lettuce, vegetables, grated cheese, salami strips and sunflower seeds topped with your dressing choice.

Baked potatoes are always topped on the side. Condiment trays featuring butter, sour cream, chives and bacon bits allow you to decide type and amount of topping. Margarine is available on request. Rice pilaf is cooked with a small amount of butter. If steamed rice is preferred allow 20 minutes and it will be cooked to order.

Two fresh vegetables are always available. Fresh vegetables come with most entrees and are served with a small amount of butter. Vegetables can be requested without fat. Vegetables (extra) may be substituted for potatoes.

Steaks are broiled. Top sirloin are 9 oz. cuts. Roasted prime rib is a 10 oz. to 11 oz. serving. Grilled chicken florentine is an 8 oz. breast serving. Salmon can be broiled and runs 7 oz. to 8 oz.

Fresh fruit may be requested at any meal. Diet beverages and artificial sweetener are available.

Mr. Herman Haastrup, executive chef, encourages his kitchen staffs to meet special needs. The same careful service and attention is given to diners just enjoying a Thunderbird/Red Lion meal as well as those staying at the motel.

*Special requests are honored with notice for Thunderbird/Red Lion banquets too.

**Trader Vic's**
**in the Benson Hotel**
**S.W. Broadway at Oak**
**Portland, Oregon**

Hours: 11:30 am–11:00 pm – closed Sunday
Reservations: Requested

Trader Vic's offers an exotic Polynesian atmosphere accented by thatched ceilings and carved masks. The cuisine is international featuring roast lamb – Indonesian style and a wide variety of Polynesian and Chinese dishes.

There is an oil and vinegar salad dressing without sugar which may be ordered to arrive on the side. The majority of the meat, poultry and seafood dishes are roasted or broiled and fresh vegetables in season are served. Most are served with the entree and vegetables may be substituted for potato. Fresh fruit or fruit juice is also available as are both butter and margarine. Baked potato topping can be served on the side and the rice is either fried or steamed depending on the dish.

Diet pop and artificial sweetener are standard. Trader Vic's serves exotic drinks from their bar and is a Portland favorite. For persons "socializing" and on a special diet they will make a non-alcoholic "Virgin Mary" – Bloody Mary's next of kin or serve soda water with a twist of lemon or lime.

Most of Trader Vic's service persons are very well informed about menu items and the kitchen is unusually good about trying to honor special requests.

**Trees Restaurant**
**Hilton Hotel**
**921 S.W. 6th Ave.**
**Portland, Oregon**

Hours: 6:30 am – 10:30 pm
Reservations: Not required
Special Menus: Childrens – Diet Entrees

The Trees Restaurant "is here to please . . . if we have it available we will prepare it" says executive chef Robert Halberg. Breakfast, lunch and dinner are served and the kitchen allows flexibility for the dieter when ordering.

Breakfast orders are available ala carte as well as in combination and eggs may be poached, boiled, toast served with butter on the side etc. Fresh fruit and unsweetened juice are available as well as a nice choice of breakfast meats and cereal.

Lunch is prepared to order so if a sandwich is your pleasure, condiments may be held or served on the side.

At dinner steak portions are 8 oz. and 10 oz. and roast prime rib is a 10 oz. serving. There are no deep fried poultry offerings and special sauces may be served on the side. Salmon and scallops are 8 oz. of broiled seafood while the sauteed trout is a 10 oz. serving.

Vegetables are included with the entree and are either fresh or frozen cooked without fat. Baked potato topping is always served on the side and the rice pilaf has not been fried or cooked in oil. Butter is served and margarine is available upon request.

Diet beverages and artificial sweetener are available, however, there is not a sugar free salad dressing.

Hilton Hotels take pride in meeting patrons' needs and The Trees Restaurant is no exception.

**Victoria Station**
**6500 S.W. Macadam Ave.**
**Portland, Oregon**

Hours: 11:30 am–2:00 pm Mon-Fri
Dinner 5:00–10:00 pm daily
Reservations: Accepted, not mandatory
Special Menus: Childrens

Victoria Station uses actual train cars for dining rooms and now offers a new menu. Many of the offerings will fit easily into a dieter's meal plan. All dinners are full meals. Lunches are available as full meals and some inflation fighters are entrees only or salad bar and soup.

The self serve salad bar is an array of fresh chopped vegetables, shirred egg, bacon bits, spinach, grated hard cheese, mushrooms, sprouts, marinated bean salad, tomatoes, beets, cucumber and seasonal vegetables. Oil and vinegar is the only sugar free dressing. The house soup is a hearty beef barley.

Prime rib is the house specialty and comes with a baked potato and your choice of salad bar or soup. The Windsor Gate cut is boneless and weighs 7 oz. to 8 oz. Track No. 1 is a boneless 11 oz. to 12 oz. serving. Track No. 2 is a hearty bone-in roast cut of 21 oz. to 22 oz.

Steaks are broiled and include top sirloin (11 oz. to 12 oz.), teriyaki beef kebob (7 oz.), teriyaki top sirloin (11 oz. to 12 oz.).

The teriyaki chicken dinner is marinated and broiled. The serving is 2 (6 oz. each) chicken breasts. (you might want to take one home in a doggie bag for lunch). The roasted duckling is approximately 1-3/4 lb. Gourmet game hens (12 oz.) are roast. The hen and duck are served with an orange sauce that may be held or served on the side.

Salmon is a 8 oz. to 9 oz. filet and will be cooked to order – broiled or poached.

Baked potatoes are routinely topped in the kitchen with your choice of butter or sour cream. On request the toppings will be served on the side so you can control the amount. The rice is steamed with a small amount of butter added. A basket of bread is served with all entrees. Butter is served with the bread. Margarine is available on request.

At lunch sandwiches can be served with condiments on the side and the hamburger is a giant broiled 8 oz. patty. The meat in the English dip is roasted and a 7 oz. prime rib cut is available.

Diet RC is served and artificial sweetener is available.

Crackers and bricks of cheddar cheese are served in the lounge area (on the house) in the evening, and the full service bar will serve non-alcoholic beverages.

Yankee Pot Roast
2839 N.W. St. Helens Road
Portland, Oregon 97210

Hours: Lunch 11:00 am–4:30 pm (Mon-Sat)
Dinner 4:30 – – – (Mon-Sat)
Sundays – Brunch 9:00am–2:00 pm – Dinner 12:00 pm – –
Reservations: Parties over 7
Special Menus: Children

The Yankee Pot Roast is a bit of real Americana. The food is 100% home made without preservatives. There are antiques throughout and the customer is really important. Families are welcome.

The bill of fare is complete dinners. For starters there is home made soup and then, green salad. The salad is tossed and topped with house dressing. The dressing has a mayonnaise base and is made without added sugar. If requested, the dressing can be served on the side.

All entrees are baked or roasted. The feature is Yankee Pot Roast and portions are approximately 6 oz. Baked ham servings run 5-1/2 oz. to 6 oz., the old fashioned roast chicken is half of a 3 lb. chicken – 1-1/2 lb. servng (includes bones). The baked meat loaf is a beef and sausage combination. There is a "pot luck" special daily.

Vegetables are included with every entree and are fresh in season or frozen. Extra vegetables may be substituted for the potato. Potatoes are boiled or scalloped. Gravy may be omitted or requested served on the side.

The hot biscuits are oversized, freshly baked and served straight from the oven with butter. Margarine is available on request.

A new dinner entree feature is a vegetable souffle. It is made from fresh eggs, bell peppers, tomatoes and cheese.

The lunch fare is pot roast, meat loaf, beef stew, a diet plate choice and chef's salad. All are served with your choice of soup or salad and the hot biscuits. At noon there are six sandwich choices (Yankee dip, meat loaf, grilled ham, cheese and tuna varieties) fixed anyway you order them! Since the customer is important, the Yankee Pot Roast will fix items to fit your needs.

Mr. Jack Ridley, creator of the Yankee Pot Roast Restaurants says "it's important to keep our customers happy. If they ask we will always do what we can." He means just that and Yankee Pot Roast Restaurants are receptive to customer requests and will try to fit your needs.

**Yaw's Top Notch**
**2001 N.E. 40th**
**Portland, Oregon**

Hours: Breakfast 7:00–11:00 am (Mon-Fri)
8:30–11:00 am (Sat-Sun)
Lunch 11:00 am–4:00 pm Daily
Dinner 5:00–12:00 pm Daily
(Burgers from 11:00 to closing)

Yaw's Top Notch has been in the Hollywood district since 1926. It is newly remodeled and the original formula hamburger, the "founder burger" is still served. The menu has expanded and includes breakfast, soup, sandwiches, steaks and seafood.

Hamburgers (founder burgers) are grilled 4 oz. patties with mayonnaise, lettuce, pickles (dill), sweet relish and your choice of tomato, cheese and onion served on a warm bun. Condiments may be omitted on request or extra dill pickles substituted for the sweet relish. The cheese and tomato are added without extra charge. Burgers come with your choice of tossed salad or French fries. A lo-cal Italian dressing is available. For the larger appetite 1/3 lb. steak size burgers are made to order.

Sandwich selections are made to order and Yaw's will dress them as requested or serve butter and/or mayonnaise on the side. Some diet popular selections include the turkey, roast beef, ham and French dip. The French dip can be requested without the sauteed onion and cheese.

The diet plate is grilled 1/4 lb. ground beef (18% average fat content), tomato wedges, peach sections, 1/2 pear, cottage cheese and 1/2 slice toasted rye bread with margarine. The fruit is canned in a sweetened syrup. Extra tomatoes may be substituted for the fruit on request.

Steaks are grilled 10 oz. filet mignon, 8 oz. and 10 oz. top sirloin, 12 oz. New York and a 5-1/2 oz. top sirloin sandwich on toast. Steak dinners include soup or salad and your choice of potato, vegetable or cottage cheese. The 8 oz. grilled halibut filet is basted with lemon butter (may be requested on the side) and served with tossed salad and choice of potato. Potatoes may be topped on the side.

Salads are available at lunch and dinner and include a chef, tuna, dinner salad, shrimp or Crab Louie. Hot vegetables are always available ala carte.

Diet pop (although not listed on the menu) is served.

Yaw's sticks to the standard menu options but many offerings have choices that will fit into a diet and any condiments can be omitted from items unless they are cooked in a special sauce.

* Take heed: Home made pies made from scratch are Yaw's special treat.

**Ye Olde Towne Crier**
**4515 S.E. 41st**
**Portland, Oregon**

Hours: 11 am – 11 pm
Reservations: Yes
Special Menus: Children and a Special "300" Meal

Home cooking and a warm atmosphere greet patrons of Ye Olde Towne Crier. Many of the customers are regulars of the Shaffer Family who make all their salad dressings, bakery items and entrees cooking from scratch.

A special diet salad dressing is served. It is made from a diet mayonnaise base and is sugar free.

A special "300" meal is served (300 denoting the calorie content) and offers a choice of broiled halibut, roast beef or broiled beef patty with two vegetables and a salad with diet dressing. The 300 is on the lunch menu and is also available at dinner if you ask. It is not listed on the dinner menu.

Ye Olde Towne Crier always tries to honor special diet requests and will always substitute cottage cheese and fruit for salad, vegies for potato and generally has fresh fruit and vegetables available. There is always a vegetable choice so it is possible to substitute an extra vegetable and have a nice variety! Vegetables are either fresh or frozen, vary seasonally and are cooked without added fats and come with most entrees.

There are many broiled and roasted meat, poultry, and seafood choices ranging from 5 oz. to 8 oz. portions. Seafood servings are generally 6 oz. All sauces may be served on the side if requested unless it is part of the cooking process.

Diet beverages and artificial sweetener are offered. Butter is served, however, margarine is available upon request. Baked potatoes are "topped" at the table as desired. The homemade rolls are served warm and butter is on the side. (The homemade blueberry jam is too but not sugar free.)

The Shaffer Family takes pride in their meals and an interest in their customers and are accomodating whenever possible. They will even take care of special needs and requests at a banquet, large group setting or on holidays if notified ahead of the occasion.

Many menu items (and lovely gifts) are available for take home at the Yankee Peddler across the street.

## WILLAMETTE VALLEY

**Al's Drive In**
**111 W. 1st Street**
**Newberg, Oregon 97132**

Hours: 11:00 am–10:00 pm daily
Reservations: No

The name Al's Drive In doesn't tell the whole story. Al's is a small clean "drive up" with limited seating and food to go and judging from the number of people on a first name basis, must be popular among the locals.

All food is cooked to order and the little place really tries to honor customers' requests and will dress the food items as you order them.

They serve the usual drive-in burgers but also have many other sandwiches (like roast beef, ham, tuna, grilled cheese), salads, pizza, spaghetti and fish and chips for starters. The soft ice cream contains 6% butter fat.

Burgers are fried patties in three size choices: 4 oz. – 2-2/3 oz. and 1.6 oz. All or any condiments may be omitted or on the side. The burger may be ordered topped as you like.

The diet plate choices are a dry tuna salad which has 4 oz. tuna, tomato slice, chopped lettuce and a piece of white toast, served daily. There is a sugar free dressing available that is made from an imitation mayo and tomato juice base. Dressing can be ordered on the side.

The other diet plate consists of 2 oz. cottage cheese, 2 tomato slices and a 4 oz. meat patty.

Al's has Tab and iced tea as well as all the usual drive-in beverages and provides artificial sweetener for the asking.

**Keg and Platter**
**3675 Market NE**
**Salem, Oregon 97301**

Hours: Lunch 11:00 am–2:00 pm
Dinner 5:00–9:30 pm
5:00–10:00 pm Fri-Sat
Reservations: Yes
Special Menus: Children

The Keg and Platter is a cordial place to meet friends or dine with your family. There are offerings that blend well into a diet and Keg and Platter will allow some substitutions.

Salad dressings can be requested on the side and there are sugar free choices with oil and sour cream bases.

Beef and seafood are featured and portions generally are 8 oz. servings. Many entrees are broiled or roasted. If broiling is your preference on an item, ask – they'll broil it. Hamburgers are always broiled. Burgers are 4 oz. and 8 oz. patties. The seafood bouillabaise is simmered.

Vegetables are varied and may be fresh, frozen or canned. Some entrees include vegetables. They are always available ala carte. Vegetables may be substituted for potatoes. Baked potatoes can be topped on the side. A 50/50 butter-margarine is used. Rice pilaf has been fried or cooked in oil.

Diet choices include ground beef with tomato, fruit or cottage cheese and a cold plate.

A vegetarian sandwich is available. All sandwiches may have condiments held or served on the side.

Fresh fruit or unsweetened fruit juice is always available.

Diet beverages and artificial sweetener are available and the bar will serve non-alcoholic beverages.

**J's Family Restaurant**
**and Pie House**
**Highway 99W**
**Monmouth, Oregon**

**J's Family Restaurant**
**and Pie House**
**At the I-5 Exit**
**Woodburn, Oregon**

Hours: 6:00 am–10:00 pm
Reservations: No

J's Restaurant and Pie House serves breakfast, soups, salads, sandwiches and full dinner meals with the whole family in mind. There are offerings for large appetites, small eaters and waist watchers.

Sandwiches include a choice of tossed salad (dressings have sour cream, mayonnaise or oil and vinegar bases), cup of soup, potato salad, or French fries. Butter, mayonnaise or any condiments may be omitted or served on the side. Good choices include ham, turkey, and French dip.

Hamburgers are fried. Patties are 3 oz. and 4 oz. servings before cooking. Burgers are served on a sesame seed bun and include tomatoes, lettuce, dressing and pickles. Condiments may be served on the side and mustard (a diet free condiment) is available on request.

Soups are home made and specials change daily. Piping hot vegetable is served daily. Soup may be ordered alone or with corn bread. (The corn bread comes with honey butter.) Plain butter or margarine is available on request.

Dinners may be ordered ala carte or as complete meals. Ala carte includes a choice of soup or salad, potato and bread and butter. Baked potatoes may be topped on the side. Vegetables may be substituted for potato. Vegetables are fresh, frozen and canned varieties without fat. A fresh vegetable plate may be requested.

Meat portions are approximately 4 oz. servings.

Waist watchers might enjoy the breast of chicken or top sirloin served with cottage cheese, fresh tomatoes and asparagus spears.

Salads are a good diet choice. Chefs salads with turkey, ham, Swiss and American cheese, egg, lettuce, and tomato are available in the regular portion or 1/2 size. Shrimp salads also have the 1/2 portion option.

J's always has fresh seasonal fruit and diet cola. Artificial sweetener is available.

J's are dependable restaurants to stop at along the road and will try to accomodate special requests within the range of their standard offerings. The menu is long, offers lots of food choices and the entire bill of fare is served from 11:30 until closing. During breakfast hours many items may be available on request.

*There are 23 home made pie specialties on the back of the menu – avoid temptation . . . read only the inside selections!

**Prime Rib Riverside**
**103 Pine N.E.**
**Salem, Oregon**

Hours: 11:30 am–2:00 pm Mon-Fri
5:30–10:00 pm Mon-Sat – Closed Sunday
Reservations: Yes

The Prime Rib Riverside specializes in beef but takes just as much pride in its fish and foul entrees. The seafood broil is a nice change of pace.

Broiled and roasted meat entrees run approximately 6 oz. to 8 oz. portions, poultry is an 8 oz. portion and fish, seafood run 8 oz. All are available not deep fried and special sauces can be held or served on the side.

Salad dressing can be omitted or served on the side and the oil and vinegar is sugar free. Vegetables are seasonal and may be fresh, frozen or canned. They are served without added fat. Some entrees include vegetables. Vegetables are always available ala carte. Vegetables may be substituted for the potato.

Baked potatoes can be topped on the side. The topping is a 50/50 butter-margarine blend. Rice is served and has been fried or cooked in oil.

Condiments, butter or mayonnaise may be held on any sandwich or requested on the side. Hamburgers are broiled and weigh 6 oz. before cooking.

There is a diet plate. It is fish or beef with cottage cheese, tomatoes, and cucumbers.

Fresh fruit or unsweetened fruit juice and artificial sweetener are available. Diet beverages are not served.

The Prime Rib Riverside makes every effort to make your dining experience a pleasure and will try to honor special requests.

**Colonial House**
**5005 Commercial, SE**
**Salem, Oregon**

Hours: 5:30 pm – 11:00 pm
Reservations: Yes
Special Menus: Childrens

The Colonial House is strictly a dinner house. Broiled and roasted meat entrees are served as are poultry and seafood specials that have not been deep fried.

Salad dressing can be served on the side. The oil and vinegar is the only sugar free salad dressing, however, fresh lemon is available.

Fresh or frozen, canned vegetables are available and not cooked with added fat and generally served with the entree.

Butter is served and margarine is available on request. Potato topping can be served on the side.

Diet beverages and artificial sweeteners are available and the bar will accomodate "non alcoholic" orders while relaxing and the kitchen will "try" to honor special needs if requested.

**The Other Place**
**2410 Mission St., SE**
**Salem, Oregon 97302**

Lunch 11 am – 2 pm
Hours: Dinner 5 pm – 10 pm –
Reservations: Yes

The Other Place does not have a deep fryer so all meat, seafood and poulty entrees are either broiled, roasted, baked, or pan fried.

Salad may be served with dressing on the side but none are sugar free. Fresh lemon is available. Vegetables are available ala carte and are frozen, canned and fresh depending on the season. However, vegetables may be substituted for the potato.

Potatoes are served with the topping on the side and a fried rice pilaf is available.

At lunch a diet plate featuring halibut or ground beef is served and broiled hamburgers are 4 oz. patties. Sandwiches may be served with garnishes on the side as requested.

Diet pop is not available, however, iced tea, unsweetened fruit juice, coffee or soda water with lemon or lime are served.

Butter, margarine, and artificial sweetener is available and the owner, John C. Wilbur, says The Other Place will try to honor special food and diet requests.

**Stuart Anderson's Black Angus Restaurant**

**2123 Franklin Blvd.
Eugene, Oregon**

**220 Commercial, SE
Salem, Oregon 97302**

Hours: Mon–Thurs 11:00 am–10:30 pm
Fri–Sat 11:00 am–11:30 pm – Sun 11:00 am–10:00 pm
Reservations: Taken
Special Menus: Childrens

Stuart Anderson's, with its western theme and private individual dining booths, features char-broiled steaks, prime rib and Alaska king crab. The restaurant attempts to accomodate most dietary needs.

The house dinner salad (now a combination of lettuce, fresh mushrooms, cherry tomato, purple onion and croutons) may be topped with two sugar free dressing choices. The blue cheese has a mayonnaise base, vinegar and oil is seasoned. Salads are included with dinner as are ranch bread (French bread topped with buttery cheese, garlic and paprika) and your choice of baked potato, French fries or rice. The rice is steamed in chicken stock without fat and the potato topping (a whipped margarine base) will be served on the side if requested. Fresh vegetables are ala carte. The potato may be substituted for cottage cheese or sliced tomatoes. (Often the cottage cheese is served on a mini pineapple slice – check with waitress to see if your particular serving is on juice or syrup packed pineapple.)

Broiled steaks at dinner are London broil 9–10 oz., filet 7-1/2-8-1/2 oz., regular cut New York and top sirloin 9–10 oz. pre cooked weight. Roast prime rib is a 9–10 oz. serving.

Alaska king crab and lobster are served steamed or baked with drawn butter on the side. Crab is an 8–10 oz. serving. Lobster tails weigh 5–6 oz.

The lunch London broil serving is 6 oz. and prime rib is 7 oz. Noon time also features a taco salad that is a bed of greens topped with 6 oz. taco meat and vegetables. Toppings are served on the side for this specialty. The taco salad is served in a large flour tortilla that has been deep fried. There are also a variety of sandwiches at noon including French dip and broiled hamburgers.

Stuart Anderson's Restaurants do a pretty good job catering to special dietary requests and their advertisment claims "It'll make you feel good inside." *Travelers note: These are part of a chain and menu is standard.

**Myrl's Chuck Wagon**
**2125 S. Pacific Blvd.**
**Albany, Oregon**

Hours: Lunch 11 am-3:30 pm — Dinner 4:30 pm-8:00 pm
Reservations: Taken for groups of 12 or more

Buffet eating out is easy on a diet as you can choose foods in the amounts you need and make choices that are tailored especially for you! Myrl's Chuck Wagon offers steamed baked chicken daily, has roast beef and various other choices; fish is generally deep fried. They have salads, vegetables (fresh, frozen, or canned depending on the season) that have been cooked without added fat.

Diet RC, tea and Postum are available as well as artificial sweetener. Butter and margarine are served.

Fresh fruit is available in season.

If you're not hungry for the full buffet meal you can choose to have salad only, or a soup, salad, drink combination.

Owner Martin Mann says they "serve an array of sugar free foods daily on the buffet line and will honor special requests whenever possible."

**Papagayo**
**550 N.W. Harrison**
**Corvallis, Oregon**

Hours: 11:30 am-2:00 pm – 5:00-9:00 pm
Reservations: Yes

Papagayo offers a straightforward collection of Mexican food choices many of which can be enjoyed on a diet and owner Randy Stern says they'll try to serve patrons with special needs "whatever they want!"

Salad seems a good place to begin and the two sugar free dressing offerings are blue cheese with a sour cream-buttermilk base and vinegar which is spicy and Spanish in nature and uses three vinegars, oil, wine and spices. Salad varieties (chef, shrimp, crab) are available.

There is a wide array of ala carte items and many savory full course dinners. The majority of the items are sauteed. Only deep fried offerings on the entire menu are tacos and chimichanga. Shrimp, snapper and crab are 4-6 oz. servings and the steak picado is an 8 oz. sirloin steak cooked in a zesty vegetable sauce. Vegetables are used throughout the Mexican offerings.

Mr. Stern noted all enchilada sauces are sugar free and have butter, spices and a bit of flour in their base. The Spanish rice has been cooked in margarine.

Sauces may be served on the side if requested and diet pop, artificial sweetener and unsweetened fruit juice are available.

Incidently, the Papagayo may be found in the form of the parrot in the colorful wall tapestry.

**Sizzler Family Steak Houses**
**General Office:**
**2101 N.W. 9th**
**Corvallis, Oregon 97330**

Hours: 11:00 am–9:00 pm
Reservations: No
Special Menus: Children

Sizzler Family Steak Houses offer a menu that is a favorite of dieters and families. The fresh vegetable salad bar is unlimited, self serve and choices may be topped with two sugarless dressings. Blue cheese dressing is a blue cheese, vinegar, mayonnaise and imitation sour cream base with special seasonings. Oil and vinegar is the second sugar free dressing.

Steaks, hamburgers and hibachi chicken are broiled. Steak cuts are 5 oz. to 10 oz. portions, chicken is a 4 oz. serving and hamburgers are 4 oz. to 8 oz. patties. The sauce for hibachi chicken may be requested on the side.

There is a choice of potato (baked or French fries), cottage cheese or rice with entrees and if none is desired, they do not charge for the potato. Margarine is served and the potato topping may be requested on the side.

Diet beverages and artificial sweetener are available.

**Mazzi's Italian Foods**
**2495 N.W. 9th**
**4250 S.E. Commercial**
**Corvallis, Oregon**

Hours: 5 – 10 pm
Reservations: Sunday – Thursday

Italian food . . . diet legal! Mazzi's has many traditional Italian offerings for your enjoyment and owner Joann Petrie says "Sugar has not been added to any of our foods. We do not cook in heavy oils. We have a range of sauces that go from delicate to thick and rich."

There are three sugar free salad dressings, thousand and blue cheese with mayonnaise for the base and a house oil and vinegar. Mazzi's features fresh crisp green salad and their calorie watchers suggestion is a Chef Salad with fresh greens, fresh mushrooms, black olives, tomato, cheese and Canadian bacon.

There is a 5 oz. roasted veal dish available and 5-6 oz. chicken portions that have been baked and sauteed. If you have any questions just ask your server to check with the kitchen.

Mazzi's pizza crusts are made from unbleached white flour with no preservatives added. They make their own pizza and spaghetti sauce daily from fresh ingredients. The minestrone soup is made with only fresh quality vegetables and flavored only with herbs and spices. (This is a great way to enjoy vegetables and eating out!) The bun bread is homemade daily, again no preservatives. Bread is served with butter on the side.

There is unsweetened apple juice, diet Pepsi and artificial sweetener available.

Soup, salad and small pasta portions may be ordered on the side. Decide your sauce and remember the pasta cooked has 70 calories (1 bread exchange) per half cup. Enjoy!

**Coburg Inn**
**209 Willamette St.**
**Coburg, Oregon 97401**
**(near Eugene)**

Hours: 11:00 am–2:30 pm - 5:00–11:00 pm
Reservations: Parties of 7 or more

The Coburg Inn Restaurant is an intimate gas lit dining room with a Victorian atmosphere in a century old house.

Meat, poultry and fish dishes are all available broiled, roasted or cooked without heavy fats. Dishes with sauce may, on request, have the sauce served on the side.

Baked potatoes can be topped on the side. Vegetables are an allowable substitution for potato and are seasonally fresh.

Fruit or unsweetened juice, diet beverages, and artificial sweetener are available.

Hamburgers are broiled and all sandwiches are made on order so condiments may be held or served on the side.

Owner Donald Savoie says the Coburg Inn will try to honor special food/diet requests of patrons.

The bar will serve non-alcoholic beverages.

**Del Taco**
**30 Country Club**
**Eugene, Oregon 97401**

Hours: 10:00 am–10:00 pm

Del Taco serves Mexican-American food, hamburgers and has a salad bar. There is dining room service after placing your order at the counter. You may drive thru the outside window and dine in your car or take food home.

Vegetables on the salad bar are fresh, canned and frozen varieties and the Italian salad dressing is sugar free. It has an oil and vinegar base. This is a favorite choice of dieters.

Sandwiches may have condiments on the side by request and hamburgers are 2 oz. patties.

Diet pop and artificial sweetener are available.

**Excelsior Cafe**
**754 E. 13th Ave.**
**Eugene, Oregon 97401**

Hours: 9:00 am–Midnight Tue-Sat
6:00 pm–Midnight Mon-Sun
Sunday Brunch 10:00 am–2:00 pm
Reservations: For Dinner

The Excelsior Cafe is located in an attractive remodeled Victorian home near the University of Oregon campus. It features a skylighted greenhouse terrace and dining room. Meals range from home made soup, salads and char-broiled hamburgers at lunch to continental evening dining. Seasonal entree specials are popular, cooked fresh and change often. Dinners may be ordered as full meals or ala carte.

Salads are available as main dishes and are included in full dinners. There are two sugar free dressings. The home made blue cheese dressing features Oregon blue cheese, mayonnaise, sour cream, herbs and spices. Vinegarette is olive and salad oils, old wine vinegar and herbs. All dressings will be served on the side if requested. Many salads are unique combinations and a nice change from ordinary restaurant fare.

Meat, fish and fowl may be charcoal broiled and lunch portions are generally 4 oz. to 5 oz. and dinner servings 6 oz. to 8 oz.

Boiled new potatoes or pasta are generally served with dinner. They may be substituted for vegetables. Vegetables are fresh, included with entrees. Some vegetables are served with butter added.

The favored hamburger is served only at lunch and on Sunday nights. The char-broiled patties are 5-1/3 oz. or 6-1/3 oz. Condiments may be omitted or served on the side of any sandwich order. Hot and cold sandwich combinations are offered.

Fresh orange and grapefruit juices are served year around and iced tea is added in the summer. Artificial sweetener is not available.

"The Excelsior Cafe rarely deep fries and never adds sugar to foods -- trying to keep things as clean tasting as possible," says manager Stephanie Pearl.

The Excelsior Cafe will honor special requests that do not disrupt the normal routine and always tries hard to please patrons.

**International Kings Table, Inc.**
**1500 Valley River Drive,**
**No. 300**
**Eugene, Oregon**

Hours: Lunch 11:00 am–3:30 pm
Dinner 4:30–8:30 pm
(International Kings Table, Inc. is part of a chain and hours may vary slightly, depending on location.)

International Kings Table restaurants are a buffet giving customers the opportunity to take any combination of foods from items offered. Food choices can generally be worked into a modified diet.

The Italian salad dressing for the do it yourself salad is sugar free. The Italian dressing base is oil, vinegar and spices.

Roast beef, baked white fish and chicken and dumplings seemingly are dieters' favorites. The gravy/sauce can not be omitted from the chicken but most can be removed when the skin is taken off.

Hot vegetables are always offered. The vegetables are seasonal and may be fresh, frozen or canned. All are served without fat.

Rolls are self serve and margarine is available.

Diet beverages and artificial sweetener are served.

Food at The International Kings Table is cooked prior to the meal time, making service rapid but menu flexibility is limited for special requests.

**Ye Olde Pancake House**
**2421 W. 11th**
**Eugene, Oregon 97402**

**Ye Ole Pancake House**
**Cottage Grove, Oregon**

**Ye Olde Pancake House**
**1060 S. Main**
**Lebanon, Oregon**

**Ye Olde Pancake House**
**1525 Franklin**
**Eugene, Oregon**

Hours: 6:00 am–10:00 pm
Reservations: Large Groups
Special Menus: Children – Senior Citizen

Ye Olde Pancake Houses serve a full days fare and tries to accomodate customer requests. Featured items include pancakes and waffles. Diet syrup is available. Whipped butter is served with items. Margarine may be requested if it fills special dietary needs.

Fresh fruit and unsweetened fruit juice are always available.

The menu includes broiled and roasted meat entrees. They are approximately 4 oz. to 5 oz. servings. Turkey is served in 3 oz. portions and seafood/fish portions are 6 oz. Any gravies or special sauces may be omitted or served on the side.

Vegetables are frozen. They are cooked and served without fat. Vegetables may be substituted for potatoes except on specials.

Sandwiches are made to order and any condiments, butter and/or mayonnaise will be held or served on the side by request. Hamburgers are broiled. Patties are 4 oz. and 5-1/3 before cooking.

There are two diet choices: Halibut or beef with cottage cheese, peach half, prune and tomatoes. The chef salad is a popular dieters choice at noon. There is not a sugar free dressing available but lemon wedges may be requested.

Diet beverages and artificial sweetener are served.

Ye Olde Pancake Houses will honor special requests and try to accomodate their customers' needs if possible. Senior citizens may even "diet out" and receive a 10% discount!

Moreno's Mexico
433 E. Broadway
Eugene, Oregon 97401

Hours: Open 4:00 pm (Tues-Sun)
Reservations: Yes
Special Menus: Children

Moreno's Mexico is located in an 1851 home and serves carefully prepared foods. The menu offers a good variety of rather adventurous items that may be worked into a modified diet. Sauces may be served on the side if requested.

The house salad dressing is a vinegar and oil base. Fresh lemons are also available. All combination dinners include tossed salad as well as a home made beef dumpling soup.

Many entrees are broiled or roasted. Carne Asada is a 12 oz. New York steak broiled Mexican style. Gallina en Mole is a 6 oz. to 8 oz. roasted chicken breast serving. Gallina is marinated in a tasty cacao bean, chile and spice sauce. Shrimp are broiled and can be ordered as an appetizer or dinner entree. Appetizers are 3 oz. to 4 oz. servings and dinner portions are 6 oz. to 8 oz. The shrimp are served with melted butter than can be held on request.

The tasty rice has been cooked with vegetable oil and butter. Vegetables are available. They are fresh or canned varieties. Vegetables are cooked and served without fat added.

Some entrees include vegetables but they are always available ala carte.

Iced tea, diet Bubble Up, diet RC and soda water are dieters' favorites. Artificial sweetner is not available.

Moreno's is a family business that has been in Eugene over 25 years. They will try to honor special requests and appreciate special requests with reservations if possible.

**Humps Restaurant**
**Columbia River Highway**
**Clatskanie, Oregon**

Hours: 6:00 am–10:00 pm
Reservations: No

Humps Restaurant serves complete meals and ala carte items all day.

Roast turkey and roast pork are 5 oz. portions and may be requested with gravies or sauce held or served on the side. Vegetables are included with most entrees. They are frozen or canned and have fat added. Baked potatoes may be topped on the side and rice has been fried or cooked in oil.

Hamburgers are 2-1/2 oz. patties that are fried and condiments may be held or served on the side. All sandwiches at Humps are made to order and may have condiments omitted or requested on the side.

The diet plate is roast beef, cottage cheese, tomatoes, egg and rye crisp. There is not a sugar free salad dressing available.

Humps serves diet beverages, artificial sweetener and fresh fruit or unsweetened juice.

If given advance notice, Humps kitchen staff will honor special diet requests.

**Pier II Feedstore**
**Restaurant & Lounge**
**77 11th Street**
**Astoria, Oregon**

Hours: 11 am – 10 pm
Reservations: Yes
Special Menus: Small Appetite

Located majestically over the Pacific, Pier II offers a full menu that is sure to please and a beautiful waterfront view.

At lunch a lovely luncheon salad bar which includes ham, turkey, cheese and approximately 17 other salad choices is available. At dinner there is also a salad bar offered with about 20 items to complement the salad basics. Their oil and vinegar dressing is sugar free.

There is a variety of meat entrees that are broiled or roasted and portion sizes run 6 oz. – 8 oz. and 12 oz. so check with your server for the size of your entree choice. The ocean's bounty is plentiful with many items not deep fried and sauces can be served on the side. Fresh broiled salmon in season is an Oregon favorite.

Vegetables are available and are canned or frozen and are served without added fat. Vegetables may be substituted for potatoes. Some entrees include vegetables but they are always available ala carte.

Butter is served and margarine is available on request. Artificial sweetener is provided and diet beverages are on the menu.

Pier II will gladly serve baked potato topping on the side and also offers a rice pilaf that has been cooked in oil.

Hamburgers are broiled and are a 4 oz. patty. Condiments will be served on the side if requested.

Relaxed, leisurely dining, a beautiful view, menu flexibility and great salad bars await you at Pier II. The bar will serve plain tomato juice or soda water with lemon or lime while you relax and socialize and the kitchen will try to honor special food/diet requests of their patrons.

Plan a few extra minutes before or after meals to browse the little shops housed in the unique warehouse building.

**The Ship Inn**
**1 -- 2nd**
**Astoria, Oregon**

Hours: 11:30 am–10:30 pm – Closed Monday
Reservations: None
Special Menus: Half Orders Available

The Ship Inn is a converted tavern – turned into a proper pub serving fresh seafood, home made sausage and Cornish and chicken pasties (English meat pies).

Seafood portions are approximately 6 oz. and some are available not deep fried. Deep fried halibut fish and chips are a house specialty.

Fresh vegetables are available and the baked potatoes can be topped with either butter or margarine on the side.

Diet beverages, fresh fruit or unsweetened juice and artificial sweetener are served.

Seafood salads and half order portions are popular with dieters and patrons with smaller appetites.

**Rob's Restaurant**
**1815 S. Holladay**
**Seaside, Oregon 97138**

Hours: 5:30 am – 8:00 pm
Reservations: No
Special Menu: Childrens

Rob's Restaurant is a good moderate priced family eating place where there's something for everyone. Rob's breakfasts seem to be a favorite of fishermen and vactioners and items can be ordered (eggs–poached – toast unbuttered – meat on the side) as needed by the patron.

Many sandwiches are available and mayonnaise, butter or any garnishes may be left off or served on the side. Hamburgers (3 oz. and 6 oz. patties) are fried. Substitutions are often allowed to fit special needs if available.

Fruit, vegetables, diet pop, artificial sweetener, butter and margarine are all on hand and Rob's makes an effort to handle special requests to the limits of their kitchen.

**Thunderbird/Red Lion**
**400 Industry Street**
**Astoria, Oregon 97103**

Reservations: Suggested
Special Menus: Children

The Thunderbird/Red Lion kitchens feature quality ingredients and flexible menus. Coffee shops and dining rooms are well stocked and make a real effort to honor special requests.

Breakfasts come in a wide range of combination plates and ala carte items. Ala carte items are easily prepared to meet special requests. Fresh fruit is always available.

Lunch and dinner menus feature offerings in a wide range in both coffee shop and dining rooms. Food is the same high quality in both kitchens with dining room service being more formal.

Soups are home made. Sandwiches may have condiments omitted or served on the side. French fries can be substituted for cottage cheese or often a cup of soup.

Blue cheese dressing is home made without added sugar and has a mayonnasie base. Vinegar and oil is also available without sugar. Lunch menus feature nice salad choices and salad (entree type) may be requested at dinner even if not on the menu. The seafood Louies have approximately 4 oz. shrimp or crab. Dinner salads are tasty combinations of lettuce, vegetables, grated cheese, salami strips and sunflower seeds topped with your dressing choice.

Baked potatoes are always topped on the side. Condiment trays featuring butter, sour cream, chives and bacon bits allow you to decide type and amount of topping. Margarine is available on request. Rice pilaf is cooked with a small amount of butter. If steamed rice is preferred allow 20 minutes and it will be cooked to order.

Two fresh vegetables are always available. Fresh vegetables come with most entrees and are served with a small amount of butter. Vegetables can be requested without fat. Vegetables (extra) may be substituted for potatoes.

Steaks are broiled. Top sirloin are 9 oz. cuts. Roasted prime rib is a 10 oz. to 11 oz. serving. Grilled chicken florentine is an 8 oz. breast serving. Salmon can be broiled and runs 7 oz. to 8 oz.

Fresh fruit may be requested at any meal. Diet beverages and artificial sweetener are available.

Mr. Herman Haastrup, executive chef, encourages his kitchen staffs to meet special needs. The same careful service and attention is given to diners just enjoying a Thunderbird/Red Lion meal as well as those staying at the motel.

**Crab Broiler**
**Highway 101**
**(3 miles south of Seaside)**
**Seaside, Oregon 97138**

Hours: Summer 11:30 am–10:00 pm
Winter 11:30 am–9:00 pm
Closed Thanksgiving & Christmas
Reservations: Suggested
Special Menus: Children and Smaller Portion

The Crab Broiler has often been featured by travel guides as one of America's outstanding roadside restaurants but the continuing popularity with travelers is the best recommendation. The menu flexibility rates 4 stars for dieters!

The Daggatt family and staff are more than willing to accomodate special needs and requests. George Daggatt stresses if customers just ask they will prepare menu items in the manner best for the patron. The spotless kitchen is well equipped to handle special preparation requests. It may take an extra few minutes for a change from the standard menu but it is well worth the wait for food cooked to special orders.

Complete dinners include the entree choice, potatoes (bakers are always served with the butter on the side), cole slaw or tossed green salad and beverage Sliced tomatoes may be substituted for the potato.

The house blue cheese dressing is sugar free and may be served on the side. Crab and Shrimp Louis – ala Crab Broiler – are available in two sizes. The large "Louis" has 6 oz. of crab or shrimp, the small 4 oz. Lemon wedges and dressing on the side are easy options. The house French bread is served with salad orders and dinners. The bread is your choice of plain, buttered, topped with whipped blue cheese, or garlic butter. The bread may also be requested toasted dry – butter on the side.

Steaks are broiled and run from a 6 oz. steak sandwich (served as a complete meal) to New Yorks (8 oz. and 12 oz.). Rib eye (8 oz. and 12 oz.) and the T-bone at 16 oz. All meat weights are uncooked.

Well prepared seafood items have long been popular. An all time Oregon favorite is the cracked dungeness crab. The whole crab weighed between 1-3/4–2 lbs. before cleaning. It is served cold and cracked ready for the diner to pick and enjoy. The crab is part of a full dinner and served with drawn butter or mayonnaise on the side. A smaller crab portion is also available. Filet of sole and halibut are 8 oz. portions and the locally caught salmon is 10 oz. Salmon, halibut and sole are delicious broiled.

The newest feature on the menu is the smaller portion features and smaller portions are served to anyone ordering them regardless of age! There are 10 smaller portion entree choices which run from seafood to chicken to pork chops! The smaller portions are perfect for the smaller appetite and dieter.

Canned vegetables (peas, beans and corn) are available on request.

Diet beverages, unsweetened orange, grapefruit, tomato and pineapple juice are served in addition to coffee, tea, Sanka, milk and skim milk. Artificial sweetener is available.

The dedicated and personal involvement of the Daggatt family with its patrons enables the Crab Broiler to meet special needs and serve the freshest seafoods available!

**Driftwood Inn**
**179 N. Hemlock**
**Cannon Beach, Oregon**

Hours: 11:00 am–10:00 pm
Reservations: No
Special Menus: Childrens, Senior Citizen

If patrons make wishes known at the Driftwood Inn the kitchen will try to accomodate special needs from the wide menu featuring salads, sandwiches, steaks and seafood.

Salad dressings may be ordered on the side and sugar free choices have oil and vinegar and sour cream bases. Salad choices include a chefs salad, Crab Louie, and slim salad. The slim salad is fresh cottage cheese, decked with assorted unsweetened fruit.

Hamburgers are broiled patties weighing 1/4 lb and 1/2 lb before cooking. Relish may be held or requested on the side. Sandwich choices include ham, beef, turkey, crab, Canadian and bacon offered in unique tasty combinations.

The broiled ground sirloin and steak cuts start at 8 oz. Clams are steamed in white wine and served with drawn butter. Broiled Pacific Coast salmon is butter brushed and may be ordered without the added butter. Full dinners include tossed salad, baked or French fried potato with an individual loaf of hot bread. Butter and margarine are available and the bread and potato may be topped on the side. Fresh sliced tomatoes will be substituted for potato on request.

Diet pop, unsweetened fruit juice and artificial sweetener are available.

On a curious note: I wonder when the extra special Hummingbird Wings are in season. When available (?) they are $18.50 and prepared to order.

**The Whaler**
**200 Hemlock St.**
**Cannon Beach, Oregon**

Hours: Noon–11:00 pm
Reservations: Summer
Special Menus: Children, Senior Citizens, Diet

The menu reads "A whaler might never put to sea if he knew he could get these fancy favorites on shore." This is right, there is something good awaiting everyone. There are choices from both land and sea.

Broiled beef steaks are 12 oz. New York cuts, filet mignon – 10 oz., top sirloin in three sizes 12 oz. – 8 oz. – 6 oz., and prime ground steaks 10 oz. Seafood favorites include scampi, salmon, halibut, prawns, oysters and Cannon Beach razor clams. Seafood entrees average 6 oz. portions. The steamed little-neck clams (a whole sand bucket full) come with drawn butter, as does the 10 oz. lobster tail.

Salad dressing may be held or served on the side. The oil and vinegar is sugar free and lemon wedges are available on request. In addition to the dinner salad, Crab Louie, Shrimp Louie (in two sizes), large tossed salad and gallery salad are served.

Full dinners include a relish dish, soup, tossed salad, choice of steamed rice or pilaf cooked in oil or potato (French fried, baked or au gratin) and bread. Baked potato topping may be served on the side and butter is served unless margarine is requested. Vegetables may be substituted for potato or rice. Some entrees have a hot vegetable (frozen) cooked without fat included.

The diet plate is 1/3 lb. broiled hamburger with cottage cheese or salad. Hamburger sandwiches are made from broiled 1/3 lb. patties. Condiments may be served on the side.

Diet beverages, artificial sweetener and fresh fruit or unsweetened fruit juices are available.

The Whaler tries to honor special patron requests and the bar will serve non-alcoholic beverages.

**Haystack House**
**Tolovania Park, Oregon**
**97145**

Hours: Winter — 11 am–3 pm and 5 pm–9 or 10 pm
Reservations: No
Special Menu: Light Eaters Portions

Haystack House is located in Tolovania Park, Cannon Beach and is open to the public as well as guests of Tolovania Inn.

Haystack House "tries to accomodate the patrons who are on special diets" and will substitute vegetables for potatoes or rice pilaf which is baked in butter. Potato topping on the side can be requested. Butter and margarine are available. The vegetables are fresh and seasonal, mostly stir fried. Some are included with entrees; others ala carte.

Either fresh fruit or unsweetened juice is always available and artificial sweetener is provided.

Salads may be served with a sugar free oil and vinegar dressing.

Meat and seafood items that are not deep fried (broiled, baked or roasted) are available and servings run from 6 to 12 oz. portions. Check with service person for more exact serving amounts.

Sandwiches can be made as you like with butter, mayonnaise or garnishes held or served on the side.

Hamburgers are broiled.

The lounge will serve non alcoholic juice and mixers on request and sugar free pop, iced tea, milk and coffee are available.

A special light eaters portion is a favorite of many dieters and is always featured and will be served to patrons of all ages!

**Hadley House**
**2203 3rd St.**
**Tillamook, Oregon**

Hours: 11:30 am–9:30 pm
Reservations: No
Special Menus: Children

The menu starts "Welcome to Hadley House" and the staff tries to meet patron needs.

The menu is flexible and begins with a self service salad bar – with or without meal. If salad is your meal choice a chef salad with lettuce, turkey, ham, cheese (Tillamook), tomato and hard boiled egg is available in two sizes. Crab and Shrimp Louies are also available – half or whole portions. The oil and vinegar is sugarless and lemon slices are also available.

Steaks are broiled and include a 5 oz. Tenderloin, 8 oz. Ground Sirloin, 8 oz. Rib Eye and 10 oz. New York. Roast beef is a favorite.

Salmon is served baked in white wine, and comes with the salad bar, choice of potato or rice which has been cooked in oil. The potato may be topped on the side. Butter is served on the table but margarine may be requested.

There are two diet corner meals. A cold plate including ham, turkey, cheese, tomatoes, rye crisp and cottage cheese. You may also choose the 3-1/2 oz. ground round patty with cottage cheese, fruit, tomatoes and rye crisp.

Hamburger sandwiches are broiled 3-1/2 oz. patties and all sandwiches may have condiments held or served on the side.

Diet beverages and artificial sweetener are available.

The luncheon menu offers patrons as many selections with as much flexibility as the dinner menu to meet modified dietary needs.

**Pixie Kitchen**
**3519 N.W. Highway 101**
**Lincoln City, Oregon 97367**

Hours: 11:30 am–8:00 pm Sun-Thu – Winter
11:30 am–9:00 pm Fri-Sat – Winter
11:30 am–9:00 pm Mon-Thu – Summer
11:30 am–10:00 pm Fri-Sat – Summer
Reservations: Advised
Special Menus Available: Childrens and Diabetic

The Pixie Kitchen is a lively family restuarant that specializes in fresh seafood, serves chicken, steaks and pork chops. The Indian style barbeque salmon is cooked over alderwood and sure to make anyone forget they're on a diet! The Pixie Kitchen is flexible and tries to be accomodating.

Dinners are available as regular or deluxe. Regular dinners include a choice of tossed salad or cole slaw, entree, garlic bread and potatoes. Salad dressing may be served on the side. Lo cal dressing is available on request. Deluxe dinners include unlimited trips to the appetizer – salad bar, entree, garlic bread and potato. Potatoes may be mashed, baked or French fried. Baked are always topped on the side. Deluxe dinners may also have entree re-orders for a nominal charge.

The salad bar has 22 dishes to select. Choices range from tossed salad, vegetable sticks, cole slaw, potato salad, bean salad and relishes to such tempting nibbles as clam dip, warm cod fish balls, crackers and cocktail bread. The salad bar can also be ordered as a meal by itself and comes with garlic bread.

Canned vegetables are always available and may be substituted for potatoes. Vegetables are served without fat added. Butter and margarine are available.

The diabetic menu is popular with persons on modified diets and includes such choices as poached cod, poached salmon, broiled sirloin and chuck steaks. Pixie Kitchen will even prepare the veal cutlets without breading on the broiler.

Fresh oranges and water packed peaches are also on the menu. Diet Pepsi, Diet 7-Up and artificial sweetener are available. The Shell Bar will serve non-alcoholic beverages.

Steaks are broiled 10 oz. top sirloin and 12 oz. New York cuts. The alder barbequed salmon is available after 5:00 pm and all day Sunday. It's a popular specialty of the Pixie Kitchen and may be ordered without the lemon-butter basting. Generous Crab and Shrimp Louies make satisfying meals and may have dressing on the side.

Hamburgers are broiled 4 oz. patties and may have condiments on the side.

Harry and Corrine Smith are specialists in family dining and will honor special requests whenever possible so the entire family may enjoy the meal . . . together. The entire menu is served all hours so there are always items for all appetites and needs.

Monday thru Saturday an all you can eat self service buffet lunch is served from 11:30 am to 2:30 pm. It features the salad bar plus 9 hot dishes that change daily. Make reservations – relax – enjoy!

**Lil Sambos Restaurant**
**3262 N.E. Highway 101**
**Lincoln City, Oregon 97367**

Hours: 6 am – 8 pm daily
Reservations: No
Special Menu: Childrens Breakfast Plate

Lil Sambos serves "breakfast" all day and lunch and dinner after 11 am. They are "primarily" a pancake house but do offer a variety that may be easily worked into a modified diet.

Juices include orange, grapefruit, pineapple, apple, prune and V8 and melon is available when in season. Bananas in cream (which may be substituted for skim milk) are a menu regular. Side order eggs, breakfast meats and toast may be ordered just the way you like or need them. There are many combination plates featuring large breakfasts as well as the standby waffle and pancakes. Assorted dry cereal, cream of wheat and oatmeal are available and may be served with skim milk. Artificial sweetener is available.

Lil Sambos will try to honor requests within the range of their kitchen and sandwiches are made to order with your choice of meat (ham, corned beef, pastrami, roast beef) and cheese (Swiss, American, or jack) on your choice of bread. Sandwiches are served with a tossed green salad. Condiments and dressing may be ordered on the side. There is not a sugar free salad dressing available.

Hamburgers are fried, 5-1/3 oz. patties, served with fries and garnished with lettuce, tomato and a relish mix that can be held or served on the side.

Dinner entrees feature two 6 oz. baked seafood items – oysters and scallops. These include all you can eat salad bar, choice of potato (baked or whipped can have topping on the side) and bread. Butter and margarine are available as is diet pop. Other items are also available, however, are generally fried or deep fried. Also offered are an all you can eat soup and salad bar after 11:00 am.

Sambos tries to cater to the whole family and make eating a pleasant experience and will try to fit your needs into the offerings; however, there is a charge for substitutions so it's often better to order ala carte choices.

**Henry Thiele's**
**at the Dunes**
**1501 N.W. 40th**
**Lincoln City, Oregon**

Hours: 7:00 am–11:00 pm daily
Reservations: Suggested
Special Menu: Children

Henry Thiele's at the Dunes is the coast branch of the long time Portland restaurant and offers a large menu, beautiful ocean view and features excellent prime rib.

The prime rib is available in three size cuts. The prime rib sandwich is approximately an 8 oz. cut of meat and is served with a tossed salad and choice of baked or French fried potatoes. The prime rib sandwich is a meal in itself and the potato condiments (butter, sour cream and chives) are always served on the side. Margarine is available on request.

The regular dinner prime rib is approximately 11 oz. and the captain's cut is 14 oz. Full dinners include your choice of clam chowder or tomato juice, a tossed salad, entree choice, potato or rice, beverage and dessert.

There is an abundant choice of grilled seafood and steak items on the dinner menu.

Fresh fruit, unsweetened juice and artificial sweetener are always available.

The lunch menu offers some flexibility as the sandwiches may have condiments held or served on the side, roast meat and salads are available, with dressing on the side. The breakfast specialty is a huge German pancake filled with butter and syrup. It can be split and one half (or both) may have the syrup held. Standard breakfast items, eggs, meat, juice, fruit and toast are available cooked as you like.

Henry Thiele's at the Dunes has been serving patrons since 1959 and will try to co-operate to special diet requests within reason.

The full service bar will serve non-alcoholic beverages. Non-alcoholic beverages are even available during live entertainment and nightly dancing hours.

**Dory Cove Restaurant**
**(Next to Road's End State Park)**
**Off Highway 101 North of Lincoln City**
**Roads End, Oregon**

Reservations: No

Dory Cove is a bit off the tourists' path but well worth finding. The restaurant is casual with a nautical decor and offers a standard menu that works well for persons on modified diets.

Diet plates and small appetite portions are regular menu features. The diet plates include broiled fish with fresh garden salad, a 4 oz. broiled beef patty with garden salad, 6 oz. broiled rib eye steak and salad or a choice of garden salad with crab or shrimp. Low calorie Catalina and Italian style dressings are available on request.

For the larger salad appetite a chefs salad, large crab and shrimp seafarers salad or combination seafarer (with dressing requested on the side) can be ordered.

Hamburgers are 1/4 lb. patties that you "build the way you want it" at the sandwich bar. These may be requested broiled.

Dinners include your choice of salad or clam chowder (very thick and rich) potato (stuffed, O'Brien or steak fries) and garlic French bread. Entrees include seafood and steaks. Broiled steaks include 8 oz. New York and top sirloin cuts, 10 oz. rib eye, a 6 oz. rib eye sandwich, and hamburger steaks. A specialty is broiled salmon. Salmon steaks and filets are available in three sizes – small (6 oz.), medium (8 oz.) and large (10 oz.) The broiled halibut steak (8 oz.) is also popular.

Diet Pepsi is the sugar free house beverage and coffee, tea (hot or cold), milk and other soft drinks are served.

Substitutions are not encouraged. The low calorie dressing can be served with any salad order.

La Plaza
4009 Highway 101 So.
(The Inn at Spanish Head)
Lincoln City, Oregon

Hours: 8:00 am–10:00 pm
Reservations: Recommended
Special Menus: Children

La Plaza is nestled in at The Inn at Spanish Head and offers a most spectacular view of the ocean and flexible menu that will fit most modified diet needs. The menu offers items from land and sea and Chef Charles Phelps will honor special food or preparation requests whenever possible.

The breakfast menu offers 12 combination meals (eggs, meats, omelettes, etc.), hot cakes, cereals and juices. Most items may be custom ordered ala carte, prepared as you choose to meet your needs in the amount desired.

Lunch features grilled halibut and salmon ( 6 oz. portions that may be requested poached or broiled), salads, an 8 oz. broiled New York steak sandwich, broiled ground sirloin with mushroom sauce and assorted hot and cold sandwiches. Sandwiches are served with your choice of ranch fries, potato salad, cole slaw or tossed green salad. The only sugar free salad dressing is vinegar and oil. Hamburgers are broiled (4 oz. or 8 oz. patties) and may have condiments served on the side. The lo cal special is 8 oz. of broiled chopped beef, cottage cheese and sliced tomatoes.

There are six broiled steak choices with cuts from 8 oz. to 12 oz. on the dinner menu and the prime rib is roasted. At dinner halibut and salmon are 8 oz. servings and may be requested broiled or poached. Shrimp and Crab Louies are available at dinner.

Vegetables are available ala carte and are seasonal. They may be fresh, frozen or canned and are served without fat added. Vegetables may be substituted for potatoes on dinner items. If a baked potato is your choice topping may be served on the side and either butter or margarine requested. Rice has been fried or cooked in oil.

Coffee, tea, Tab, Sanka and milk are served. Tomato, unsweetened orange and grapefruit juice are available.

**Salishan Lodge**
**Gourmet Room**
**Sun Room**
**Gleneden Beach, Oregon**

Hours: Sun Room – 7:00 am–8:30 pm
Gourmet Room – 6:00 pm –
Reservations: Gourmet Room only

Salishan will honor special requests, particularly if advance notice can be given. In the Gourmet Room this is easiest done at the time of reservation, however, there are many diet "legal" items on the regular menu.

The special French, Salishan salad dressing is sugar free, tasty and may be served on the side. In figuring calories it has an oil and lemon juice base.

There are many broiled and roasted entree offerings and beef portions run 8 – 10 – 12 and 16 oz. Check with the waiter for the size of your serving if you have questions. The chicken breast (a low fat entree) is an 8 oz. portion. Seafood and fish items not deep fried include sole, cod, salmon, crab and shrimp. Seafood portions are 6-8 oz servings.

Salishan always has vegetables available and 95% of them are fresh. Generally vegetables are served with butter but the butter can be omitted on request and a lemon wedge substituted. Baked potato topping also can be served on the side. If the rice pilaf is your choice add a fat exchange to allow for that oil used in preparation.

Diet beverages are available as well as artificial sweetener.

Butter is the house standard, however, if requested, margarine may be substituted.

The Sun Room offers a full days fare and has fresh fruit and unsweetened fruit juice available all hours and special breakfast and lunch items may be ordered ala carte. On sandwiches butter, mayonnaise or other garnishes may be held or served on the side. The hamburgers are grilled and patty sizes before cooking are 5 oz. and 8 oz. portions.

The dining room has an "on the light side" page with offerings that are a favorite with "diet watchers."

If socializing, the lounge has diet soda, iced tea and is most willing to serve soda water with a lime, or plain tomato juice for your relaxation and enjoyment.

Salishan restaurants are open and welcome both guests and non-guests of the lodge.

**Marketplace Restaurant**
**Gleneden Beach, Oregon**

Hours: 11:30 am–9:00 pm
Reservations: No

The Marketplace Restaurant is located in the Salishan Shopping Mall. It's rapidly gaining in popularity among residents and tourists. The menu has a limited selection but if the Marketplace can do anything for special diet requests they will.

Broiled main entrees are available. The New York steak is a 10 oz. cut. Tasty broiled halibut is a 8 oz. to 10 oz. serving.

Hamburgers are broiled 5-1/3 oz. patties and any condiments may be requested held on the side. All menu sandwiches are made to order and special requests honored.

Baked potatoes and canned vegetables are not available. Rice pilaf is served and has been fried or cooked in oil.

There is a nice fresh fruit plate in season with yogurt or cottage cheese. Crab and shrimp salads are also on the menu.

Diet Pepsi is served and artificial sweetener is available.

Casey's
Agate Beach Hilton
3019 North Coast Highway
Newport, Oregon 97365

Hours: 7:00 am–11:00 am – 11:30 am–2:00 pm –
5:30 pm–9:00 pm daily
Reservations: Yes
Special Menu: Childrens

Casey's at the Agate Beach Hilton offers an ocean view and carefully prepared food. In true Hilton style Casey's will try to honor special requests.

The dinner menu features fresh salmon in season (Chinook or silver) cooked to your request, poached, broiled or baked and a nightly fish choice fresh from the docks prepared your choice of poached, broiled or fried. In season a house specialty is boiled crawfish. Fish specialties are served with vegetable and potato. There are a variety of seafood specialties as well ranging 6-8 oz. portions. Vegetables are seasonally fresh or frozen and cooked without added fat. Soon to be added to the regular menu is a vegetable main dish variety. Vegetables not presently included with dinner may be ordered ala carte.

Potato butter may be served on the side and the rice is prepared without oil.

Meat items are varied and combinations of steak and seafood can be ordered. Roast and broiled meat portions range 6-10 oz. at dinner, 4-5 oz. at lunch.

Diet beverages, artificial sweetener, and fresh fruit are available.

The oil and vinegar dressing is sugar free and menu substitutions are not generally allowed.

The full service bar will serve non-alcoholic beverages.

House of Almerik
121 So. Pacific Way
Newport, Oregon 97365

Hours: 4:30 pm–1:00 am
Reservations: Only (1-503-867-6841)
Special Menus: Childrens, Senior Citizens, Diet

The House of Almerik serves meals made to order. This small restaurant serves fresh, carefully prepared food that you order when making the reservation.

The owner-chef, John McKern says "each person should pre order their dinner at time of reservations allowing unlimited selection and cooking instructions for dietary meals."

This restaurant is special as it is true — Chef McKern will prepare anything within reason. Service and atmosphere are only second to the highest quality of food!

Salads may be dressed with two sugar free dressings, blue cheese with a mayonnaise base and a special 1000 island with mayonnaise, fresh pineapple and papaya blended with tomato sauce and seasonings.

All steaks are top broiled and choices run from a 6 oz. New York or filet to a 10 oz. filet, 12 oz. sirloin and New York cuts. The roast prime rib is available cut in 8 oz., 12 oz. or 16 oz. portions.

The special Chicken Kiva is a 7 oz. breast. All seafood entrees are sauteed, baked or poached. Entrees might include snapper, ling cod, salmon, sole, halibut, crab, oysters, scampi, prawns or razor clams cooked to your individual taste. Most seafoods are 7 oz. portions.

Baked potatoes come with entrees and are always topped on the side. Choose toppings and amount from butter, sour cream, chives and bacon bits.

Vegetables are available and may be cooked without added fat by steaming or boiling.

Diet beverages, fresh fruit, unsweetened juice and artificial sweetener may be requested.

The choices are flexible and almost endless. The hardest part is deciding what to order! Relax and enjoy Almerik!

**Neptune's Wharf Restaurant**
**665 N.W. Nye**
**Newport, Oregon 97365**

Hours: 11:00 am – 9:00 pm
Reservations: Suggested
Special Menus: Childrens

Make reservations for a window table and not only enjoy your meal but the view of Newport Bay with seals at play, the fishing fleet and sailing ship Sara.

Seafood is the house specialty and there are many items not deep fried. The large steamed scampi are served in shells with drawn butter on the side. There are also steamed butter clams, lobster and scallops sauteed with vegetables to name a few. Bouillabaisse with green salad is always a treat. Steaks are broiled and come in 8 oz. and 13 oz. cuts. With your entree you can choose a steamed rice pilaf, baked potato and request condiments on the side or sliced tomatoes or steamed zucchini may be substituted. Vegetables are fresh and prepared without added fat. Salads may be topped with two sugar free dressings, roquefort with a mayonnaise–buttermilk base and oil and vinegar. If plain sour cream or lemon slices only is your choice for salad topping, they are available. In addition to the dinner salad the menu offers Crab and Shrimp Louies, Chefs Salad and a fresh fruit salad.

Many sandwich choices are offered and are made to order so condiments may be held or on the side. Butter is served. Hamburgers are grilled 4 oz. patties.

The luncheon Bayside diet plate is a hamburger patty, sliced tomatoes, cottage cheese and hot cheese bread.

Diet beverages are not served; however, iced tea, coffee, milk and unsweetened fruit juice are available. Artificial sweetener is provided.

Neptune's Wharf offers a full menu with a wide range to choose from and will try to honor special dietary requests to the best of their ability.

**Whales Tale Inc.**
**452 S.W. Bay Blvd.**
**Newport, Oregon 97365**

Hours: Mon-Th 7 am-8 pm — Fri-Sat 9 am-10 pm — Sun 9 am-7 pm
Reservations: No

The Whales Tale is located amidst the bustle of the Newport bay front and offers some sound diet choices.

Beginning with breakfast there are omelette combinations offered with hearty home fries and a homemade muffin, but the most diet conscious way is the "side orders" which feature poached eggs, ham, sausage and toast or a homemade bagel that can be ordered with the butter on the side. Bagels may also be topped with your choice of cream cheese, tomatoes, onion and sprouts. Orange juice, apple juice, coffee and tea are available but not artificial sweeteners. Diet Pepsi is on the menu as is mineral water.

Hamburgers are a 6 oz. patty that is grilled and mayonnaise and condiments can be omitted or served on the side.

Dinners include salad and the spicy oil and vinegar and blue cheese in a sour cream base are both sugar free. White fish may be ordered poached or grilled and is a 7-8 oz. serving. Potatoes are a nice change in small boiled reds.

And co-owner Kathleen Kelly-Schwartz suggests the white fish, seafood salad or Chefs Salad in place of the traditional "diet plate."

Non meat eaters might find the vegeburgers made from a soybean and rice base to their liking.

There are a variety of sandwiches offered as well and Ms. Kelly-Schwartz says the Whales Tale will make substitutions to fit special needs whenever possible and even cook special requests "when we're not very busy!"

**The Experience**
**3750 Highway 34**
**Waldport, Oregon**

Hours: Open 5:00 pm Wed-Sat – Sundays open 3:00 pm
Reservations: Yes

The Experience Restaurant serves carefully prepared seafood only, stressing no short cuts and nothing battered or deep fried.

Full dinners only are served and "your entree choice can be baked or poached when the quality will not be impaired," states partner Janice Willinger. Unless requested otherwise all items are prepared with fresh butter. Dinners include appetizer (usually crudite with aioli) soup, salad, entree, steamed red skin potato, warm sourdough bread and hot tea or coffee.

There are two sugar free salad dressings. Green Goddess has a sour cream and mayonnaise base. The roquefort is made with IMO and buttermilk.

Portion sizes are generous. Halibut is 8 oz., steamed clams weigh 2 pounds in the shell, lobster tails are 8-10 oz., scampi are 8 oz. and scallops and prawns are 1/3 pound before breading. Each item is prepared to order in its own individual pan. Clams are steamed with white wine, celery and herbs. Dungeness crab legs are poached in white wine boullion and served with drawn butter.

Diet soda is not available but Perrier water is offered year around and in the summer iced tea and coffee are added to the menu.

**Manni's Hilltop House**
**116 North Bay Drive**
**North Bend, Oregon 97459**

Hours: 5:00–11:00 pm – Mon-Sat
5:00–9:00 pm – Sun
Open Holidays
Reservations: Suggested
Special Menus: Young Friends and Not So Hungry

Manni's Hilltop House sits high above Coos Bay revealing the panorama of water and dunes to the end of the horizon. The food and special handling of requests is equally impressive.

Dinners are served with a choice of Boston clam chowder or tossed salad, a baked potato, French fries or rice pilaf and garlic bread or rolls.

All Manni's salad dressings are made without added sugar and generally have a mayonnaise base.

The rice pilaf has a small amount of margarine added. Potatoes can be topped on the side.

Veal is a house specialty. Portions average 4 oz. and are cooked in butter. Veal choices include classic dishes from Italy, Switzerland, Austria and France. Sauces may be served on the side.

The Bouillabaisse is a tureen of shrimp, crab legs, butter clams, snapper, scallops, halibut and prawns that have been simmered in a wine and herb broth. This tasty special broth has only a very small amount of salad oil per serving. Bouillabaisse is served with green salad, garlic bread and a bib!

Steaks are broiled and feature New York (16 oz. and 12 oz.), filet mignon (12 oz. and 8 oz.), and top sirloin (6 oz., 8 oz. and 12 oz.).

Salmon is an 8 oz. portion and broiled fresh in season. Salmon "monte carlo" is poached and served with an egg yolk rich hollandaise that can be ordered on the side. Many other seafood offerings can be requested broiled. Vegetables are always available.

Manni's will take special care in preparing food to meet dietary needs. The kitchen is most cooperative and will take the extra time to prepare items right and do special requests justice. The staff is flexible and takes pride in doing the extra for their patronage.

**Thunderbird/Red Lion**
**1313 N. Bayshore Drive**
**Coos Bay, Oregon 97420**

Reservations: Suggested
Special Menus: Children

The Thunderbird/Red Lion kitchens feature quality ingredients and flexible menus. Coffee shops and dining rooms are well stocked and make a real effort to honor special requests.

Breakfasts come in a wide range of combination plates and ala carte items. Ala carte items are easily prepared to meet special requests. Fresh fruit is always available.

Lunch and dinner menus feature offerings in a wide range in both coffee shop and dining rooms. Food is the same high quality in both kitchens with dining room service being more formal.

Soups are home made. Sandwiches may have condiments omitted or served on the side. French fries can be substituted for cottage cheese or often a cup of soup.

Blue cheese dressing is home made without added sugar and has a mayonnasie base. Vinegar and oil is also available without sugar. Lunch menus feature nice salad choices and salad (entree type) may be requested at dinner even if not on the menu. The seafood Louies have approximately 4 oz. shrimp or crab. Dinner salads are tasty combinations of lettuce, vegetables, grated cheese, salami strips and sunflower seeds topped with your dressing choice.

Baked potatoes are always topped on the side. Condiment trays featuring butter, sour cream, chives and bacon bits allow you to decide type and amount of topping. Margarine is available on request. Rice pilaf is cooked with a small amount of butter. If steamed rice is preferred allow 20 minutes and it will be cooked to order.

Two fresh vegetables are always available. Fresh vegetables come with most entrees and are served with a small amount of butter. Vegetables can be requested without fat. Vegetables (extra) may be substituted for potatoes.

Steaks are broiled. Top sirloin are 9 oz. cuts. Roasted prime rib is a 10 oz. to 11 oz. serving. Grilled chicken florentine is an 8 oz. breast serving. Salmon can be broiled and runs 7 oz. to 8 oz.

Fresh fruit may be requested at any meal. Diet beverages and artificial sweetener are available.

Mr. Herman Haastrup, executive chef, encourages his kitchen staffs to meet special needs. The same careful service and attention is given to diners just enjoying a Thunderbird/Red Lion meal as well as those staying at the motel.

*Overnight guests may also have special items requested via room service.

**Jot's Resort**
**North End – Rogue River Bridge**
**Highway 101**
**Wedderburn, Oregon 97491**

Hours: 7:00 am–10:00 pm daily
Reservations: Suggested
Special Menus: Light Suppers

Jot's Resort is located on the lower end of the Rogue River. From the dining room one can enjoy seals and sea lions playing in the harbor and bay. Food is carefully prepared and special requests are honored whenever possible. The new light suppers are favorites of dieters and people with smaller appetites. The menu is most informative and tells portion size and preparation method of each item.

Seafood and steak entrees include a fresh relish tray, choice of soup or salad, baked potato, rolls and coffee. Salads may be topped with a sugar free home made blue cheese dressing or a combination of vinegar and olive oil. Potatoes may always be topped on the side.

Vegetables are always available. Some entrees include cooked vegetables, other vegetables are ala carte.

Salmon is an 8 oz. serving and can be grilled or poached on request. Fresh red snapper is a 6 oz. portion. A 7 oz. scallop specialty is marinated in special wine sauce with button mushrooms, skewered and broiled. Steaks are char grilled to order. Cuts range from a 6 oz. top sirloin to a 10 oz. New York.

Diet beverages and artificial sweetener are available.

From the food service Anne Arntzen says Jot's will do their best to handle special requests. She asks patrons to allow a few extra minutes for special preparation. Jot's wants your visit to be just right and realizes the importance of special dietary needs and guests with questions or special requests can phone ahead.

After a day of salmon fishing, riding the Rogue or beach combing it's nice to relax and know Jot's will accomodate special meal requests.

**Tad's Chicken 'n' Dumplings**
**U.S. Scenic Highway 30**
**Troutdale, Oregon**

Hours: 5:00 pm-1:00 am Mon-Sat
2:00-11:00 pm Sun
Reservations: No
Special Menus: Childrens

Tad's Chicken 'n' Dumplings has been a landmark on the bank of the Sandy River for over 30 years. Informal, it's a good family restaurant.

The house specialty is chicken and dumplings. The dinner is a large bowl of boiled chicken and two dumplings in tasty gravy. The chicken can be requested without the gravy or with the gravy on the side. It is a 10 oz. to 12 oz. chicken portion. Salad (oil and vinegar dressing is sugar free), rolls (butter and margarine are available), vegetable, coffee and dessert come with the meal.

Vegetables are canned. They are cooked and served without added fat.

Tad's also offers grilled salmon and steaks. There is a sandwich selection. Hamburgers are fried 4 oz. patties. Condiments on all sandwiches may be held or served on the side.

The menu also includes three dinner salads, chicken, shrimp and crab.

Diet beverages, fruit juice and artificial sweetener are available.

Tad's is busy and one can expect to wait, especially during the summer. Drinks are served on the outdoor patio (under cover) and non-alcoholic beverages are available.

**Forest Inn**
**54737 E. Highway 26**
**Sandy, Oregon 97055**

Hours: 5:30–10:30 pm
Reservations: Recommended
Special Menus: Children and Special Requests

The menu has printed the following: For the gourmet who desires favorite or unusual dishes, **we invite and welcome special requests.** This applies to persons on special diets, vegetarians, and the general public. Substitutions are allowed.

Forest Inn serves complete dinners with home made soup, tossed salad, baked potatoes or rice, home made individual loaves of bread, desserts and beverage.

There is a sugar free salad dressing that is home made with oil, vinegar and spices. Vegetables are fresh or frozen and included with entrees. Extra vegetables may be substituted for the potato or rice. Rice has been steamed without fat. Potatoes may be topped on the side.

Butter is served and margarine is available on request for the bread. (If you don't finish your loaf, ask for a doggie bag. The left over bread makes great toast or fancy little sandwiches.)

Most meat entrees are grilled with olive oil. They range in size from 5 oz. to 12 oz. The prime rib (Friday, Saturday and Sunday) is roasted and a 15 oz. cut. The Chicken Kiev is a house specialty. It is a baked 7 oz. chicken breast. Chicken Kiev, Royal Hawaiian features the stuffed breast of chicken, served in one half fresh pineapple with a bed of rice. Interesting and surely not a typical diet meal! Sauces can always be requested on the side.

Salmon (8 oz.) is baked or poached. The hollandaise can be requested on the side. A herb sauce is served with the baked seafood (8 oz.) combination plate.

Diet beverages, artificial sweetener, fresh fruit and unsweetened juice are always available. The bar will serve non-alcoholic beverages.

Entrees are carefully prepared. Richard Estes, owner/maitre'd, encourages patron requests, and does his best to accomodate special needs.

Chalet Swiss
Highway 26
Welches, Oregon 97067

Hours: 5:00 pm Wed-Sun – Closed Mon-Tues
Reservations: Recommended
Special Menus: Children – Vegetarian

Chalet Swiss abounds with friendly atmosphere, authentic Swiss decor and costumes and food carefully prepared under the watchful eye of owner-chef Curt Mezger. Fresh, first quality ingredients are used for the cooked to order meals.

The menu has items that cater to a diet and the relaxing atmosphere and good food make it well worth the trip.

All entrees include homemade daily soup, tossed salad and a basket of freshly baked "Buerli." The buerli are tender rolls, crispy on the outside and soft inside. They are worth saving a bread exchange for and are served with butter. Margarine is available on request.

The salad is offered with two sugar free dressing choices: The House, a refreshing light oil, lemon and herb combination and blue cheese with a sour cream–mayonnaise base. Soup changes daily and ranges from warm thick cream soups in the winter to refreshing chilled summer soups.

Fresh vegetables are served with entrees and have been cooked in butter. Baked potatoes are available and the topping can be served on the side or the potato and butter cooked rice substituted for extra vegetables.

Broiled salmon is a 7 oz. portion and the light and right entree is 5 oz. of veal escallops topped with mushrooms and served with three fresh vegetables. The medallions of beef can be ordered without the sauce. An 8 oz. filet mignon and 10 oz. New York steak are offered broiled and the bearnaise sauce may be requested served on the side.

Perrier water, iced tea, hot tea, and coffee and artificial sweetener are available.

Cocktails are served at the table and may include the above beverages, plain tomato juice or soda water with lime.

Good appetizers might include the fromage, fruit – assorted imported cheeses served with fresh fruit or Buenderfleisse, a paper thin dried beef.

**Timberline Lodge**
**Dining Room on Mt. Hood**
**above Government Camp,**
**Oregon**

Hours: 6:00-9:00 pm
Reservations: Yes
Special Menus: Low Sodium Item — Vegetarian Item

The Timberline Lodge dining room sticks primarily to standard items but offers choices a person on a modified diet can enjoy after a day in the snow.

Broiled and roasted meat entrees are available. Portions run 6 oz. to 9 oz. The sauteed chicken breast is a 6 oz. serving. Sauces can be held or served on the side. Non deep fried fish and seafood items run 4-6 oz. per serving.

Fresh vegetables are also available and come with most entrees. Vegetables are seasonal and may be requested without added fat. Vegetables may be substituted for potatoes. Potatoes may be topped on the side. Butter is served. Rice pilaf has been fried or cooked in oil. Tossed salad is served and dressing may be held or served on the side. Dressings served are not sugar free.

Fresh fruit or unsweetened fruit juice are always available.

All sandwiches may have condiments held or served on the side. Hamburgers are broiled and patties are 3.2 oz. before cooking.

Diet beverages and artificial sweetener are available. The lounge will serve non-alcoholic beverages.

**Timberline Lodge Cafeteria**

The cafeteria opens daily at 8:00 am and serves self service cafeteria fare until 5:00 pm. When night skiiing is on the cafeteria is open until around 8:00 pm. This seems to be a popular place with families and dieters as you can pick and choose the foods you desire and it is also quick and informal.

**Kah-Nee-Ta**
**Warm Springs Indian Reservation**
**Warm Springs, Oregon 97761**

Hours: 7:00 am – – –
Reservations: Please

Kah-Nee-Ta is as popular with people seeking a day in the sun and a swim in the warm pools or those who stay a day or two leisurely enjoying the warmth, golf, view of restful hills and babbling warm springs river. Persons with special dietary needs can relax – Kah-Nee-Ta lodge is exceptionally good about honoring any special request they can. Kah-Nee-Ta has two eating areas at the lodge that will serve meals to lodge and non lodge guests.

The **Pinto Room** is more than the standard resort coffee shop as special requests are honored and the menu is flexible. The Pinto Room serves breakfast, lunch and dinner. Breakfast items are available ala carte or as plate meals. There egg omelettes are featured and may be "filled" on request with your choice of diet legal ham, cheese, onion and mushrooms. Omelettes are served with toast that can be requested dry with the butter on the side.

Fresh fruit and unsweetened juice are always available.

Lunch varieties can be easily modified or worked into a diet plan. Sandwiches may have any condiments omitted or served on the side. Most cold sandwiches are served with butter or mayonnaise so check and request what's best for you. Cold sandwich choices include ham and cheese, roast beef, turkey, corned beef, and club. The club can be made without the middle bread on request. Sandwiches are on your choice of bread and served with French fries, cole slaw or potato salad. I've even had them substitute a cup of soup for the accompaniment when it fit my dietary needs.

Salads include rolls and butter on the side and there is a sugar free dressing. The sugar free dressing has an Italian oil and vinegar base. Vegetable salad choices include a chef's, Shrimp or Crab Louie and stuffed tomato with chicken or tuna filling. A beautiful fresh fruit plate is available seasonally and is served with cottage cheese or sherbet. (The sherbet has 120 calories per half cup and equals 1 bread – 1 fat exchange.)

Hamburgers are broiled 5-1/3 oz. patties. Condiments may be requested on the side. Cole slaw, French fries or potato salad come with burgers, but sliced tomatoes may be substituted. A broiled rib-eye steak sandwich is also available at noon.

Lunch items are available on the dinner menu. The ground sirloin is an 8 oz. broiled portion topped with mushroom sauce. The sauce may be requested on the side. This is accompanied by tossed salad, choice of potato (may be topped on the side), vegetable, roll and butter. Vegetables are fresh or frozen – cooked and served without added fat.

The Waist Watcher is 1/3 lb. broiled ground beef, cottage cheese, sliced tomatoes, and 1 slice of whole wheat or rye toast served dry.

Diet pop and artificial sweetener are available.

The **Juniper Room** is a dinner house and reservations are needed.

Meat, fish and poultry entrees can be roasted, poached, or broiled and sauces can be requested on the side. The salmon is always fresh and excellent broiled with the dill sauce on the side. Salmon portions are 8 oz. to 9 oz. Steaks are broiled and run 10 oz. to 14 oz.

The Kah-Nee-Ta clay bird is a house specialty and must be ordered with the reservation. It is a boneless game hen, stuffed with dressing and wrapped in clay. The hen is baked in the clay and you get the fun of cracking it at the table (waitress brings a mallet). This is served with a huckleberry sauce on the side.

Dinners include soup, mixed green salad, choice of potato or rice pilaf and Indian fry bread.

Potatoes may be topped on the side and the rice pilaf is cooked and served without added fat.

The Italian vinegar and oil base dressing is sugar free. Sometimes raw vegetable relishes are served. Cooked vegetables are cooked without fat and are fresh or frozen varieties. Many entrees include vegetables (check with server) and vegetables are available ala carte.

The Indian fry bread is deep fried and much like eating a doughnut (especially with the huckleberry jam). It may be substituted for a roll on request.

The Juniper Room serves two traditional Indian dinner salads. The Ri Sho Shay is salmon, crab and shrimp, avocado and tomato wedges on fresh greens with asparagus spears, eggs and radish rosettes. The Wau Lu Kas Salpawit is the camp feast salad. This is a fresh salad for anyone and is chunks of salmon, roast beef, ham and turkey mingled with hard boiled eggs and cheese. This comes with sliced tomatoes and green onions on a bed of fresh greens. Dressing may be requested on the side and salads are served with a roll and butter.

Fresh fruit and unsweetened juice, diet beverages and artificial sweetener are always available.

The bar and lounge areas will serve non-alcoholic beverages.

Mr. Jack Daniels, food and beverage director, says Kah-Nee-Ta gladly will honor any special request they can – and he means it!

*Occasionally special requests take an extra bit of time because of the large numbers served but they are worth waiting for.

*If you have special medical needs and are a lodge guest – request a room with refrigeration

**Original Joe's**
**1033 Northwest Bond**
**Bend, Oregon**

Hours: 11:00 am–12:00 pm Mon-Thurs
11:00 am–2:30 am Fri
5:00 pm–2:30 am Sat
5:00 pm–11:00 pm Sun
Reservations: Suggested

Original Joe's makes everyone feel welcome – almost at home. The kitchen has a unique open policy that encourages patrons to order foods that meet their needs.

Fresh, quality ingredients are used. Soups, sauces and various offerings are home made. Specialties are Italian style featuring chicken and veal.

The kitchen will answer any preparation and portion questions. Owner David Merrifield thrives on happy guests. If you need your chicken skinned and baked – just ask – it may take a few extra minutes but will be prepared as ordered.

Original Joe's is unique. The personal attention, carefully prepared foods and fair prices make Original Joe's a must for individuals with special needs and a treat the entire family will enjoy.

Beef and Brew Bend
3194 North Highway 97
Bend, Oregon 97701

Hours: 5:00–10:00 pm
Reservations: Yes
Special Menus: Childrens

Beef and Brew offers various grilled steaks, seafood choices and chicken. Dinners are complete with French bread, tossed salad and your choice of cottage fries or rice pilaf. The rice pilaf has been baked in a buttery broth.

The bread and salad are the first course and butter and salad dressings are on the side. The salad arrives family style for self serve and none of the dressings are sugar free. Oil and vinegar is available as are lemon slices if requested.

Grilled steaks can be ordered from 7 oz. – 12 oz. sizes (check with server for size of your cut choices), and the prime rib is roast. The broiled chicken breast is an 8 oz. serving and may be served without sauce or with the sauce on the side. Fish and seafood entrees are 6 oz. – 8 oz. portions. Cod and scallops are deep fried, scampi is sauteed in butter and lobster tails are broiled.

Baked potatoes are available ala carte with condiments always served on the side.

Beef and Brew tries to be flexible within limits of the menu and if your server is aware of your needs, they will try to be most helpful. Beef and Brew is easy to fit into your dietary needs as so much of the food comes plain to be dressed at the table.

Seating is in booths in an arena surrounding a large fireplace. Dinners can also be ordered to include beverages as an option. Diet beverages and artificial sweetener are available.

**The Tumalo Emporium**
**64619 Highway 20 W.**
**Bend, Oregon**

Hours: 11:30 am–11:00 pm
Reservations: Yes
Special Menus: Childrens – Vegetarian

The Tumalo Emporium has an 1800's decor, features brass, red velvet and antiques along with a mahogony bar from a Nevada ghost town.

The Tumalo Emporium serves full lunch and dinner buffets plus menu choices. Owner Ann Rasmussen says the buffet is a favorite with dieters because "they may select foods of their choice." Roast beef is a buffet feature as are vegetables, prepared various ways.

Both butter and margarine are available as are diet beverages and artificial sweetener. Fresh fruit or unsweetened juice are also on hand.

The regular menu includes original house specialties, seafood and steaks. Seafood entrees are approximately 6 oz. portions and none have been deep fried. Poultry entrees are 6 oz. portions and all have special sauces that can be served on the side. Baked potato or rice comes with most dinners and potato topping can be served on the side. The rice pilaf has been fried or cooked in oil.

Several dinner salads are offered and come with a cup of homemade soup and fresh homemade bread. Salads to choose from include Crab Louies, Chefs Salad, assorted salad plate, garden salad and chicken salad. There is not a sugar free dressing; however, oil and vinegar or lemon is available on request.

If an item requested is available and not part of your order, substitution is possible. Some do, however, have an extra charge.

The luncheon diet plate is cottage cheese, tomato and ground beef patty.

The Tumalo Emporium is family owned and operated, and features fresh, home-cooked quality ingredients prepared in a variety of ways. The wide range of offerings make it possible to accomodate most dietary needs. With advance notice the kitchen will attempt to prepare items using methods other than menu standard.

**Blue and White Cafe**
**1825 Main**
**Baker, Oregon 97814**

Hours: 6 am-8 pm Monday thru Saturday. Closed Sunday
Reservations: No

The Blue and White Cafe is "like eating at home" says owner Edward Brehmer and they do not buy any cooked or pre-seasoned food.

They will try to honor special diet requests and all meats, poultry and seafood are not deep fried. In fact the Blue and White Cafe doesn't even have a deep fryer! Great for dieters! Entrees include vegetables (may be canned, frozen, or fresh depending on the season) without added fats.

Diet beverages, artificial sweeteners, and fresh fruit or unsweetened fruit juice is available. Margarine is served.

Upon request potato topping, sandwich garnishes and salad dressings can be served on the side or omitted. Extra vegetables may be also substituted for potato.

**The Rangler**
**Family Steak House**
**1914 Adams Avenue**
**LaGrande, Oregon 97850**

Hours: Weekdays 11 am — 10 pm — Sunday 12 Noon — 9 pm
Reservations: Yes
Special Menu: Childrens

At the Rangler begin dinner with the self serve salad bar. The oil and vinegar dressing is sugar free and on Sundays they offer a special dinner that is usually roasted or broiled.

The Rangler is mainly a steak house with a variety of cuts and sizes, but also does serve poultry (sauce can be requested on the side) and non deep fried seafood entrees that are approximately 5 oz. portions.

Fresh, frozen, canned, and seasonal vegetables are available cooked without added fat and extra vegetables may be substituted for the potato. Baked potato topping is always served on the side. The rice pilaf has been cooked in the oven with butter added. Butter and margarine are served.

The Rangler will try to cook foods as requested, has fresh fruit or unsweetened fruit juice available as well as diet beverages and artificial sweetener.

**Thunderbird/Red Lion**
**Highway I-84N & 11th**
**Pendleton, Oregon 97801**

Reservations: Suggested
Special Menus: Children

The Thunderbird/Red Lion kitchens feature quality ingredients and flexible menus. Coffee shops and dining rooms are well stocked and make a real effort to honor special requests.

Breakfasts come in a wide range of combination plates and ala carte items. Ala carte items are easily prepared to meet special requests. Fresh fruit is always available.

Lunch and dinner menus feature offerings in a wide range in both coffee shop and dining rooms. Food is the same high quality in both kitchens with dining room service being more formal.

Soups are home made. Sandwiches may have condiments omitted or served on the side. French fries can be substituted for cottage cheese or often a cup of soup.

Blue cheese dressing is home made without added sugar and has a mayonnasie base Vinegar and oil is also available without sugar. Lunch menus feature nice salad choices and salad (entree type) may be requested at dinner even if not on the menu. The seafood Louies have approximately 4 oz. shrimp or crab. Dinner salads are tasty combinations of lettuce, vegetables, grated cheese, salami strips and sunflower seeds topped with your dressing choice.

Baked potatoes are always topped on the side. Condiment trays featuring butter, sour cream, chives and bacon bits allow you to decide type and amount of topping. Margarine is available on request. Rice pilaf is cooked with a small amount of butter. If steamed rice is preferred allow 20 minutes and it will be cooked to order.

Two fresh vegetables are always available. Fresh vegetables come with most entrees and are served with a small amount of butter. Vegetables can be requested without fat. Vegetables (extra) may be substituted for potatoes.

Steaks are broiled. Top sirloin are 9 oz. cuts. Roasted prime rib is a 10 oz. to 11 oz. serving. Grilled chicken florentine is an 8 oz. breast serving. Salmon can be broiled and runs 7 oz. to 8 oz.

Fresh fruit may be requested at any meal. Diet beverages and artificial sweetener are available.

Mr. Herman Haastrup, executive chef, encourages his kitchen staffs to meet special needs. The same careful service and attention is given to diners just enjoying a Thunderbird/Red Lion meal as well as those staying at the motel.

## SOUTHERN OREGON

**Chata**
**1212 So. Pacific Highway**
**Talent, Oregon**

Hours: Summer 5:00-9:30 pm daily
Winter Thu-Sun 5:00-9:30 pm
Reservations: Appreciated
Special Menu: Young People's Portions

A side trip to Chata, the little house on the old highway to Ashland, is worthwhile. Chata is a little cottage in Poland and the Eastern European heritage of the Slowikowski family is reflected in the menu.

The food served features high quality ingredients that have been lovingly prepared and contain little or no added fat or sugar. The black board changes weekly and always features a cooked to order fresh poached fish dish (8 oz.), an entree of beef or pork that is roast or in a stew (beef pot roast 6-8 oz., pork roast 6-8 oz.) and a baked chicken (3/4 lb. with bone) prepared in an ethnic style. There is also a meatless dish of an East European country.

The regular menu features many specialty items. The sausage for dinner (5-6 oz.) is a choice of smoked Polish or Hungarian sausage served with boiled potato and dinner vegetables. The lamb shank (3/4 lb. with bone) is marinated in a herb marinade and served with broiled vegetables on a bed of gryka (parsley rice) that has not been fried or cooked in heavy oils. This is accompanied by Baklazhannaia Ikra "eggplant caviar." All specialty items on the menu are as interesting as those mentioned above.

A tureen of hot home made soup with tossed salad and home baked bread is popular and soups are prepared with fresh stocks and vegetables. Generally there is a choice of meat or non meat soup.

House dressings for salad are all home made and sugar free. Choices include a lemon herb, yogurt cheese and parsley mayonnaise. Dressing can be served on the side.

Vegetables come with entrees and are fresh, cooked and served without added fat. Vegetables may be substituted for potato. Butter is served on the side for bread, potato or vegetables.

Apple juice is always available and fresh fruit is usually offered in the summer. Beverages (sugarless) include coffee, tea, milk, club soda and Perrier water. Artificial sweetener is generally available.

Chata offers good food, friendly service and tries to honor special requests. A stop at Chata adds special charm to a trip to the Shakespearian Festival and is one of the most unique restaurants in the Rogue Valley.

**Beef and Brew Roseburg**
**2060 Stuart Parkway**
**Roseburg, Oregon**

Hours: 5:00–10:00 pm
Reservations: Yes
Special Menus: Childrens

Beef and Brew offers various grilled steaks, seafood choices and chicken. Dinners are complete with French bread, tossed salad and your choice of cottage fries or rice pilaf. The rice pilaf has been baked in a buttery broth.

The bread and salad are the first course and butter and salad dressings are on the side. The salad arrives family style for self serve and none of the dressings are sugar free. Oil and vinegar is available as are lemon slices if requested.

Grilled steaks can be ordered from 7 oz. – 12 oz. sizes (check with server for size of your cut choices), and the prime rib is roast. The broiled chicken breast is an 8 oz. serving and may be served without sauce or with the sauce on the side. Fish and seafood entrees are 6 oz. – 8 oz. portions. Cod and scallops are deep fried, scampi is sauteed in butter and lobster tails are broiled.

Baked potatoes are available ala carte with condiments always served on the side.

Beef and Brew tries to be flexible within limits of the menu and if your server is aware of your needs, they will try to be most helpful. Beef and Brew is easy to fit into your dietary needs as so much of the food comes plain to be dressed at the table.

Seating is in booths in an arena surrounding a large fireplace. Dinners can also be ordered to include beverages as an option. Diet beverages and artificial sweetener are available.

**Yankee Pot Roast**
**720 N.W. Sixth Street**
**Grants Pass, Oregon 97526**

Hours: Lunch 11:00 am–4:30 pm (Mon-Sat)
Dinner 4:30 – – – (Mon-Sat)
Sundays – Brunch 9:00am–2:00 pm – Dinner 12:00 pm – –
Reservations: Parties over 7
Special Menus: Children

The Yankee Pot Roast is a bit of real Americana. The food is 100% home made without preservatives. There are antiques throughout and the customer is really important. Families are welcome.

The bill of fare is complete dinners. For starters there is home made soup and then, green salad. The salad is tossed and topped with house dressing. The dressing has a mayonnaise base and is made without added sugar. If requested, the dressing can be served on the side.

All entrees are baked or roasted. The feature is Yankee Pot Roast and portions are approximately 6 oz. Baked ham servings run 5-1/2 oz. to 6 oz., the old fashioned roast chicken is half of a 3 lb. chicken – 1-1/2 lb. servng (includes bones). The baked meat loaf is a beef and sausage combination. There is a "pot luck" special daily.

Vegetables are included with every entree and are fresh in season or frozen. Extra vegetables may be substituted for the potato. Potatoes are boiled or scalloped. Gravy may be omitted or requested served on the side.

The hot biscuits are oversized, freshly baked and served straight from the oven with butter. Margarine is available on request.

A new dinner entree feature is a vegetable souffle. It is made from fresh eggs, bell peppers, tomatoes and cheese.

The lunch fare is pot roast, meat loaf, beef stew, a diet plate choice and chef's salad. All are served with your choice of soup or salad and the hot biscuits. At noon there are six sandwich choices (Yankee dip, meat loaf, grilled ham, cheese and tuna varieties) fixed anyway you order them! Since the customer is important, the Yankee Pot Roast will fix items to fit your needs.

Sunday brunch is served from 9:00 am–2:00 pm and overlaps with dinner. If part of your party wants brunch and other members dinner, that's super. Home made croquettes are a special feature, but if pot roast better fits your needs – just say so. Yankee Pot Roast people will gladly provide the pot roast.

Mr. Jack Ridley, creator of the Yankee Pot Roast Restaurants says "it's important to keep our customers happy. If they ask we will always do what we can." He means just that and Yankee Pot Roast Restaurants are receptive to customer requests and will try to fit your needs.

| The Skinny Spot | The Thinnery |
|---|---|
| 218 S.W. G Street | 259 Barnett Road |
| Grants Pass, Oregon | Medford, Oregon |

Both The Skinny Spot in Grants Pass and The Thinnery in Medford, Oregon cater to people with special dietary needs. Their customers consist of diabetics, high blood pressure patients, those with low blood sugar, dieters and others that are just interested in good nutrition.

Everything served is portion controlled and nothing is fried. They serve no beef or ham meals as the owners have found that a person who has to limit these items usually wants to save them for a special time or have them in a dinner house restaurant. They also have counts for everything served. Many products have no added sugar or sodium. These are featured in both locations.

On the things that they prepare to order, such as the salads (with sugar free dressing), pocket sandwiches and the baked fish, the salad dressings, imitation mayonnaise or the sauce can be served on the side.

The Skinny Spot and The Thinnery also carry Skinny Haven dinners, salad dressings and Skinny Munchies. These are all portion controlled, however, they do have added sodium. Recently both locations started carrying Dieters Gourmet salad dressings, pudding and whipped topping mix.

Although hamburgers are not served most children also enjoy the meals. For anyone owner Nancy Driskell says she "will be happy to split an item in such a way that they could eat part of it and take the other part home for another meal."

Fresh vegetables are available as are 8 kinds of diet beverage, fresh fruit and unsweetened juices.

Menu samples include: Thick Crust Pizza, Veal Lasagna, Veal Stuffed Peppers, Chicken Enchilidas.

All of the items are available also to take home and freeze.

Also featured is a rather complete line of cookbooks for all of their "special people."

All of The Skinny Spot and The Thinnery employees have had to use a special diet, for one reason or another. This has really helped them to have an understanding staff.

Mrs. Driskell says "We have had many rewarding experiences serving people with special dietary needs and I think in the future you will see more and more restaurants following our lead." Both restaurants are a dieters "haven" – enough said – Enjoy!

**Sir Loin**
**525 Stevens St.**
**Medford, Oregon 97501**

Hours: 11:00 am–9:00 pm
Reservations: No
Special Menus: Children, Diet

Sir Loins is a good family restuarant offering many items that can work into a modified diet. Steaks are flat grilled and there is a nice self serve salad bar. The salad bar can be a meal itself or as an ala carte addition to any meal.

The house blue cheese salad dressing is sugar free. It is prepared from a mixture of mayonnaise, buttermilk, IMO, vinegar, blue cheese and spices. Oil and vinegar and fresh lemon are also available. The salad bar is large and offers fresh broccoli, cauliflower, carrots, tomatoes, eggs, kidney beans, alfalfa sprouts, peas, barley, beets (not pickled), croutons, bacon bits, sunflower seeds and corn relish. The corn relish has added sugar. There is also a bowl of home made potato salad and occasionally cole slaw.

Beef steaks (top sirloin) are available in 6 oz. – 8 oz. – 12 oz. – 16 oz. cuts. The ground beef dinner is 8 oz. The ham steak is 6 oz. and liver and onions an 8 oz. serving. These dinners all include a baked potato or fries and roll. Margarine is served and potatoes may be topped on the side. Cottage cheese, tomato or canned pineapple may be substituted for potato.

The steak sandwich is a 4 oz. portion and burgers are 4 oz. and 8 oz. patties. The menu selection also offers many other sandwich varieties. All sandwiches may have condiments omitted or served on the side. Half sandwich, soup combos are served.

Deep fried seafood and chicken items are on the menu. Maui Chicken is a special and consists of a 4 oz. chicken patty, 1 oz. ham slice, 1 oz. Swiss cheese slice and pineapple ring.

Most items on hand may also be purchased as side orders. Portions such as 3 oz. thinly sliced turkey, 4 oz. steak, 4 oz. ham, 4 oz. cheese, 2 oz. ham and 2 oz. cheese combo, 4 oz. fish patty, and 4 oz. chicken patties are available. Side orders with the salad bar and a roll make good meal combinations.

Diet Pepsi, iced tea, coffee, tea, milk and buttermilk are served. Artificial sweetener is available.

The Sir Loin staff will honor special requests whenever possible. The wide range of combinations available make it possible to accomodate most any diet needs.

**Thunderbird/Red Lion**
**200 N. Riverside**
**Medford, Oregon 97501**

Reservations: Suggested
Special Menus: Children

The Thunderbird/Red Lion kitchens feature quality ingredients and flexible menus. Coffee shops and dining rooms are well stocked and make a real effort to honor special requests.

Breakfasts come in a wide range of combination plates and ala carte items. Ala carte items are easily prepared to meet special requests. Fresh fruit is always available.

Lunch and dinner menus feature offerings in a wide range in both coffee shop and dining rooms. Food is the same high quality in both kitchens with dining room service being more formal.

Soups are home made. Sandwiches may have condiments omitted or served on the side. French fries can be substituted for cottage cheese or often a cup of soup.

Blue cheese dressing is home made without added sugar and has a mayonnasie base. Vinegar and oil is also available without sugar. Lunch menus feature nice salad choices and salad (entree type) may be requested at dinner even if not on the menu. The seafood Louies have approximately 4 oz. shrimp or crab. Dinner salads are tasty combinations of lettuce, vegetables, grated cheese, salami strips and sunflower seeds topped with your dressing choice.

Baked potatoes are always topped on the side. Condiment trays featuring butter, sour cream, chives and bacon bits allow you to decide type and amount of topping. Margarine is available on request. Rice pilaf is cooked with a small amount of butter. If steamed rice is preferred allow 20 minutes and it will be cooked to order.

Two fresh vegetables are always available. Fresh vegetables come with most entrees and are served with a small amount of butter. Vegetables can be requested without fat. Vegetables (extra) may be substituted for potatoes.

Steaks are broiled. Top sirloin are 9 oz. cuts. Roasted prime rib is a 10 oz. to 11 oz. serving. Grilled chicken florentine is an 8 oz. breast serving. Salmon can be broiled and runs 7 oz. to 8 oz.

Fresh fruit may be requested at any meal. Diet beverages and artificial sweetener are available.

Mr. Herman Haastrup, executive chef, encourages his kitchen staffs to meet special needs. The same careful service and attention is given to diners just enjoying a Thunderbird/Red Lion meal as well as those staying at the motel.

*Overnight guests may also have special items requested via room service.

**The Dairy Queen**
**231 Redwood Highway**
**Cave Junction, Oregon**

Hours: 10:00 am–8:30 pm

The Dairy Queen at Cave Junction offers a good respite before or after touring the Oregon Caves. Although the food menu is limited they will try to honor special requests.

Sandwiches may be served with any condiments omitted or you may request specific condiments when ordering. All sandwiches are made to order. Hamburgers are grilled and patties are 2 oz. and 3.2 oz. before cooking.

Fresh fruit or unsweetened fruit juice is available.

Diet beverages and artificial sweetener for coffee are standard features.

**White Rhino**
**Wildlife Safari**
**Winston, Oregon**

Hours: 9:00 am–5:00 pm Winter
9:00 am–6:00 pm Summer
Reservations: No

Wildlife Safari offers a simple bill of fare that will fit well into a diet plan. A ticket thru the wildlife area is good for two trips on the day purchased so often it is fun to make a day of it at Wildlife Safari.

Sandwiches are the mainstay of the menu. Roast beef, ham and turkey are 2-1/2 oz. portions. Hamburgers are 4 oz. char broiled patties. All condiments may be held or served on the side. Hot dogs can be requested in the microwave.

Tomato, unsweetened orange and apple juice are always available.

Diet Pepsi and artificial sweetener is available. Diet Pepsi is also available at the outside snack area but foods that best accomodate a special diet are from the main White Rhino restaurant.

**Oregon Caves Chateau**
**Oregon Caves National Monument**
**Oregon Caves, Oregon 97523**

Hours: 7:00 am-8:30 pm
Reservations: Yes
Special Menus: Children, Vegetarian on request

A trip to the intriguing Oregon Caves is complete with a visit to the Chateau, a beautiful old wooden lodge. The Chateau is nestled in a ravine and surrounded with traditional Oregon greenery and small animals. The dining room is cheerful and has a babbling mountain stream running through. The chef goes the extra miles to meet special needs.

Meals are traditional with European style cuisine. All items can be prepared without much grease or coatings. Many items can be baked or steamed. Chef Arthur G. Axelson says "dining should be pleasurable and the food edible and nutritional." He also adds that all rolls, soups, dressings, etc. are prepared entirely from scratch!

Mr. Axelson has the knowledge and is willing to design special diet meals on request to meet individual needs. His kitchen is generally well stocked to honor special requests.

Salads may be topped with sugarless oil and vinegar or fresh lemon wedges and vegetables can be substituted for potato. Potatoes are always topped on the side. Butter is served. Margarine can be obtained on request. Rice pilaf has a small amount of oil added.

Meat entrees are generally grilled but could be baked in the convection oven without grease or coating. Portions average 6 oz. to 8 oz. Roast turkey is available in 6 oz. to 8 oz. servings.

Trout (6-8 oz.) can easily be grilled without flour or butter. Salmon filets are delicious baked or steamed.

Vegetables are always available and can be served without fat. They are seasonal and may be fresh, frozen or canned. The Chateau also features a vegetarian plate on request.

Fresh fruit is available in season and unsweetened juice is always stocked.

Tab and iced tea are served in addition to other beverages. The lounge will serve non-alcoholic drinks.

Oregon Caves is a most interesting place to visit. Your trip can be so relaxing with a night in the peaceful surroundings of the lodge and diet perfect meals in the Oregon Caves Chateau Restaurant. The restaurant hosts hotel guests and non-hotel patrons. Chef Axelson makes everyone welcome and does his best to make your visit one to remember . . . because your meals were right!

Special attention is given to requests of patrons at breakfast, lunch and dinner. Items may be purchased ala carte or condiments held or requested on the side.

**North's Chuck Wagon**
**3600 South 6th**
**Klamath Falls, Oregon 97061**

Hours: Lunch 11:00 am-4:00 pm – Dinner 5:00-8:30 pm
Reservations: No
Special Menu: Childrens

At North's Chuck Wagon you can tailor your meal to the buffet line offerings to meet your needs.

The baron of beef has been roasted and is probably the easiest meat to work into a diet. Most seafood and poultry items are deep fried.

There is always a salad variety, however, none of the dressings are sugar free.

Vegetables are always available and are fresh, frozen, canned and seasonal varieties. They are cooked and served without added fat. Margarine is available if you wish.

Diet beverages, coffee, tea, milk and artificial sweetener are served.

The buffet line features all you can eat – so take what you want. Flexibility varies as do the buffet offerings and since food is pre cooked, preparation options are unavailable. The self serve buffet offers ready meals at moderate prices.

## FAST FOODS

### Burger King Restaurants

Burger King food items are prepared to order and can be dressed to your liking. Any standard condiment can be held by request.

Burgers are broiled and Burger King serves diet pop.

Mr. Paul Dwyer of the area franchise office shared the following caloric information. Mr. Dwyer added many dieters save calories by omitting the mayonnaise. Real mayonnaise is used and all size/ variety of Whoppers contain 1/4 oz. mayonnaise.

| | |
|---|---|
| Hamburger | 290 calories |
| Cheeseburger | 350 calories |
| Whopper | 630 calories |
| Whopper w/cheese | 740 calories |
| Whopper Junior | 370 calories |
| Whopper Jr. w/cheese | 420 calories |
| Fish Sandwich | 584 calories |
| French Fries | 210 calories |
| Onion Rings | 270 calories |

### Burgerville USA

Burgerville colossal burgers are dressed to order. Patties are fresh, grilled 1/4 lb. and 1/2 lb. servings before cooking. Standard condiments include cheese, tomato, lettuce, pickle, ketchup, special sauce (a mayonnaise, mustard and relish combination) on a sesame seed bun. All or any condiments may be omitted on request.

Baked ham and cheese sandwiches contain approximately 2-1/4–2-1/2 oz. lean sliced ham and approximately 1 oz. of cheese. Ham and cheese are dressed with the special sauce (above) but may have the sauce omitted. Cheese can also be omitted if your preference is a plain ham sandwich.

Some Burgerville locations now offer a self serve salad bar. When offered the sald bar is available in the small (one serving) size or large (all you can eat) size and is an interesting assortment of lettuce, fresh sliced mushrooms, chopped egg, cheese, tomato, peas, cucumber slices, beets, garbanzo beans, sprouts and sunflower seeds. Low calorie salad Italian dressing and vinegar and oil are dieters' best choices.

Tab is served. Artificial sweetener is not available.

## KENTUCKY FRIED CHICKEN

*These figures are approximate as chickens vary in size and shape.

| Item | Calories | g/edible serving wt. Protein | Fat | Carbohydrate |
|---|---|---|---|---|
| Original Recipe | | | | |
| Wings | 136 | 9.6 | 9.0 | 4.2 |
| Drumsticks | 117 | 12.1 | 6.5 | 2.6 |
| Ribs | 199 | 16.2 | 11.7 | 7.1 |
| Thighs | 257 | 18.4 | 17.5 | 6.5 |
| Keels | 236 | 23.9 | 12.3 | 7.4 |
| Extra Crispy | | | | |
| Wings | 201 | 11.2 | 13.5 | 8.7 |
| Drumsticks | 155 | 13.3 | 9.0 | 5.1 |
| Ribs | 286 | 17.2 | 17.8 | 14.1 |
| Thighs | 343 | 20.4 | 23.4 | 12.6 |
| Keels | 297 | 23.6 | 16.4 | 13.6 |
| KFC Potatoes | 62.9 | 1.5 | 0.9 | 12.2 |
| KFC Gravy | 23.0 | 0.4 | 1.8 | 1.3 |
| Potatoes and Gravy | 85.9 | 1.9 | 2.7 | 13.5 |
| KFC Rolls | 60.6 | 1.8 | 1.1 | 10.9 |
| Corn (2-3") | 91.9 | 2.5 | 1.5 | 17.0 |
| (4-5") | 169 | 4.6 | 2.8 | 31.2 |
| Cole Slaw | 121.9 | 0.9 | 7.5 | 12.7 |
| *Original Recipe 2 pc dinner No. 1 (wing & rib + extras) | 603.7 | 30.4 | 32.1 | 48.3 |
| No. 2 (wing & thigh + extras) | 661.8 | 32.6 | 37.8 | 47.8 |
| No. 3 (drum & thigh + extras) | 643 | 35.1 | 35.2 | 46.2 |
| Extra Crispy 2 pc dinner No. 1 (wing & rib + extras) | 755 | 33.0 | 42.6 | 59.9 |
| No. 2 (wing & thigh + extras) | 812.4 | 36.2 | 48.2 | 58.4 |

*Dinners consisted of 2 pieces of chicken, with potatoes and gravy, cole slaw and a roll.

## NUTRITIONAL COMPOSITION – TACO BELL MENU ITEMS

**TACO** (159 cal.) (3 oz.)

| | |
|---|---|
| Moisture | 63.7% |
| Protein | 12.2 |
| Fat | 10.7 |
| Carbohydrates | 10.6 |
| Minerals | 2.8 |
| | 100% |

**PINTOS 'N CHEESE** (231 cal.) (7 oz.)

| | |
|---|---|
| Moisture | 71.8% |
| Carbohydrates | 12.4 |
| Protein | 6.2 |
| Fat | 5.7 |
| Minerals | 3.9 |
| | 100% |

**NCHIRITO** (391 cal.) (7-3/4 oz.)

| | |
|---|---|
| Moisture | 63.5% |
| Carbohydrates | 12.5 |
| Protein | 10.6 |
| Fat | 9.5 |
| Minerals | 3.9 |
| | 100% |

**BEEFY TOSTADA** (232 cal.) (6-3/4 oz.)

| | |
|---|---|
| Moisture | 68.8% |
| Carbohydrates | 11.8 |
| Protein | 9.3 |
| Fat | 7.8 |
| Minerals | 2.3 |
| | 100% |

**TOSTADA** (206 cal.) (5-1/2 oz.)

| | |
|---|---|
| Moisture | 71.3% |
| Protein | 9.7 |
| Carbohydrates | 10.1 |
| Fat | 5.9 |
| Minerals | 3.0 |
| | 100% |

**BEAN BURRITO** (345 cal.) (6-1/2 oz.)

| | |
|---|---|
| Moisture | 57.7% |
| Carbohydrates | 26.0 |
| Protein | 7.4 |
| Fat | 6.0 |
| Minerals | 2.9 |
| | 100% |

**LLBEEFER** (243 cal.) (5-1/4 oz.)

| | |
|---|---|
| Moisture | 62.3% |
| Carbohydrates | 19.4 |
| Protein | 9.1 |
| Fat | 5.5 |
| Minerals | 3.9 |
| | 100% |

**BURRITO SUPREME** (387 cal.) (8-1/2 oz.)

| | |
|---|---|
| Moisture | 67.7% |
| Carbohydrates | 15.8 |
| Protein | 7.4 |
| Fat | 7.0 |
| Minerals | 2.1 |
| | 100% |

The **Taco Bell** Restaurants in **Salem, Bend, Corvallis** and **McMinnville** have shared the following information:

Sauces and toppings may be omitted on request.

Diet Pepsi and artificial sweetener are available. 100% ground beef is used and as part of the cooking process excess fat is drained off.

Taco Bell will allow any omissions and certain extra ingredients may be added for a small charge.

## McDONALD'S
## OREGON LOCATIONS

2910 Newburg Road
Woodburn, Oregon 97071

2048 N.E. 3rd St.
Bend, Oregon 97701

511 N.E. Garden Valley
Roseburg, Oregon 97470

3303 Broadway Ave.
North Bend, Oregon 97459

1691 N. Hwy. 99W
McMinnville, Oregon 97128

245 Barnett Road
Medford, Oregon 97501

1891 N. 6th St.
Grants Pass, Oregon 97256

1140 Biddle Road
Medford, Oregon 97501

12090 S.W. Main
Tigard, Oregon 97223

12005 N. Center
Portland, Oregon 97217

1550 E. Burnside
Gresham, Oregon 97030

1874 Avalon Blvd.
Klamath Falls, Oregon 97601

3315 Pacific Ave.
Forest Grove, Oregon 97116

1110 Center St., S.E.
Salem, Oregon 97301

4020 Commercial St., S.E.
Salem, Oregon 97302

1101 Lancaster Dr., N.E.
Salem, Oregon 97301

2250 S.W. 9th St.
Corvallis, Oregon 97330

1320 N. 1st
Hermiston, Oregon 97837

1315 W. 6th
The Dalles, Oregon 97058

900 Southgate
Pendleton, Oregon 97801

820 S.W. Alder
Portland, Oregon 97205

9475 Beaverton Hillsdale
Beaverton, Oregon 97005

3519 Cedar Hills
Beaverton, Oregon 97005

559 S.E. 10th Ave.
Hillsboro, Oregon 97123

551 N.E. 122nd Ave.
Portland, Oregon 97230

1831 W. Burnside
Portland, Oregon 97209

3232 E. Pacific
Albany, Oregon 97321

1580 Coburg Road
Eugene, Oregon 97401

2250 S. Main
Lebanon, Oregon 97355

2308 Island City Hwy.
LaGrande, Oregon 97850

55 River Ave.
Eugene, Oregon 97402

1417 Villard Ave.
Eugene, Oregon 97403

1565 Mohawk Blvd.
Springfield, Oregon 97477

1300 N. Coast Hwy.
Newport, Oregon 97365

6300 N. Lombard
Portland, Oregon 97203

3330 N.E. 82nd
Portland, Oregon 97220

10151 S.W. Capitol Hwy.
Portland, Oregon 97219

2875 S.E. Powell Blvd.
Portland, Oregon 97202

9100 S.E. Powell Blvd.
Portland, Oregon 97266

18430 S.E. Stark
Portland, Oregon 97233

15114 S.E. McLoughlin Blvd
Milwaukie, Oregon 97222

1979

## REVISED DIABETIC FOOD EXCHANGE LIST FOR McDONALD'S® RESTAURANTS

To assist persons following diabetic diets, listed below is exchange unit information for food served at McDonald's.

| | Exchange Units | Calories | Cholesterol (mg) |
|---|---|---|---|
| **Hamburger** | 2 bread, 1 high fat meat | 260 | 25 |
| **Cheeseburger** | 2 bread, 1½ high fat meat | ,300 | 40 |
| **Quarter Pounder®** (wt. before cooking ¼ lb.) | 2 bread, 3 high fat meat | 420 | 70 |
| **Quarter Pounder with Cheese** | 2 bread, 4 high fat meat | 520 | 95 |
| **Big Mac™** | 2½ bread, 3 high fat meat, 1½ fat | 540 | 75 |
| **Filet-O-Fish™** | 2½ bread, 1½ lean meat, 3½ fat | 400 | 45 |
| **French Fries** (regular) | 1½ bread, 2 fat | 210 | 10 |
| **Egg McMuffin®** | 2 bread, 2 high fat meat, 1 fat | 350 | 190 |
| **Pork Sausage** | 1 high fat meat, 1½ fat | 180 | 45 |
| **English Muffin** buttered | 2 bread, 1 fat | 190 | 10 |
| **Hash Browns** | 1 bread, 1½ fat | 130 | 10 |
| **Scrambled Eggs** | 1½ medium fat meat, 1 fat | 160 | 300 |
| ***Hot Cakes with Butter & Syrup** | 4 bread, 3 fruit, 2 fat | 470 | 35 |
| ***Chocolate Shake** | ½ skim milk, 3½ bread, 2 fat | 360 | 30 |
| ***Vanilla Shake** | ½ skim milk, 3 bread, 1½ fat | 320 | 30 |
| ***Strawberry Shake** | ½ skim milk, 3½ bread, 1½ fat | 340 | 30 |
| ***Apple Pie** | 1 bread, 1½ fruit 3½ fat | 300 | 15 |
| ***Cherry Pie** | 1 bread, 1½ fruit 3½ fat | 300 | 15 |
| ***McDonaldland® Cookies** | 3 bread, 2 fat | 290 | 10 |
| ***Sundaes** | | | |
| **Hot Fudge** | 2 bread , ½ whole milk, 1 fruit, 1 fat | 290 | 20 |
| **Strawberry** | 1 bread, ½ whole milk, 2 fruit | 229 | 20 |
| **Carmel** | 2 bread , ½ whole milk, 1 fruit | 282 | 20 |
| **Pineapple** | 1 bread, ½ whole milk, 2 fruits | 230 | 20 |

*These items contain sucrose sugar. Persons with diabetes are strongly discouraged from eating items in which significant carbohydrate is derived from sugar. This carbohydrate is quickly absorbed resulting in an abrupt peaking of the blood sugar.

## WENDY'S INTERNATIONAL, INC.
## OREGON LOCATIONS

1560 Pacific S.E.
Albany, Oregon 97321

1609 N.E. 3rd St.
Bend, Oregon 97701

925 So. Broadway
Coos Bay, Oregon 97420

2300 N. 9th St.
Corvallis, Oregon 97330

1965 River Road
Eugene, Oregon 97404

2830 Willamette St.
Eugene, Oregon 97405

1895 Franklin Blvd.
Eugene, Oregon 97403

2401 W. 11th St.
Eugene, Oregon 97402

1829 N.E. 6th
Grants Pass, Oregon 97526

490 E. Burnside
Gresham, Oregon 97030

955 S.W. Oak
Hillsboro, Oregon 97123

2323 S 6th
Klamath Falls, Oregon 97601

1730 N. Highway 99W
McMinnville, Oregon 97128

940 S. Riverside
Medford, Oregon 97501

17217 S.E. McLoughlin
Milwaukie, Oregon 97222

256 East Idaho Ave.
Ontario, Oregon 97914

824 Southgate
Pendleton, Oregon 97801

16220 S.E. 82nd Drive
Portland, Oregon 97266

1405 No. Lombard
Portland, Oregon 97220

232 N.E. 82nd Ave.
Portland, Oregon 97220

4829 S.E. 82nd Ave.
Portland, Oregon 97266

5226 S.W. Beaverton Hills
Portland, Oregon 97221

615 S.E. 122nd
Portland, Oregon 97233

798 N.W. Garden Valley
Roseburg, Oregon 97470

641 Lancaster Dr., N.E.
Salem, Oregon 97301

2375 S. Commercial St.
Salem, Oregon 93702

1499 Mohawk St.
Springfield, Oregon 97477

12785 S.W. Pacific Highwa
Tigard, Oregon 97223

## DIABETIC FOOD EXCHANGE LIST FOR WENDY'S RESTAURANTS

**The information listed below is for those people who are on restricted or diabetic diets. The sandwich items include ketchup, mustard, mayonnaise, onions, pickles, lettuce and tomatoes.**

| Item | Exchange Units | Calories | Cholesterol (mg) | Sodium (mg) |
|---|---|---|---|---|
| Single | 2 bread, 3 lean meat, 3 fat | 470 | 70 | 774 |
| Double | 2 bread, 6 lean meat, 4 fat | 670 | 125 | 980 |
| Triple | 2 bread, 9 lean meat, 5 fat | 850 | 205 | 1217 |
| Single Cheese | 2 bread, 4 lean meat, 4 fat | 580 | 90 | 1085 |
| Double Cheese | 2½ bread, 6 lean meat, 6 fat | 800 | 155 | 1414 |
| Triple Cheese | 2 bread, 10 lean meat, 7 fat | 1040 | 225 | 1848 |
| Chili | 1½ bread, 2 lean meat | 230 | 25 | 1065 |
| French Fries | 3 bread, 3 fat | 330 | 5 | 112 |
| *Frosty | 4 fruit, 1 whole milk, 1 fat | 390 | 45 | 247 |

*This item contains sucrose sugar. People who have diabetes are strongly discouraged from eating items in which significant carbohydrate is derived from sugar. This carbohydrate is quickly absorbed, resulting in an abrupt peaking of the blood sugar.

**Wuvs**
**Beaverton, Oregon**

**Wuvs**
**S.E. 82nd and King Road**
**Portland, Oregon**

**Wuvs**
**Gresham, Oregon**

**Wuvs**
**Clackamas Town Center**
**Clackamas, Oregon**

Wuvs serves breakfast, burgers, fried chicken, chili, a salad bar and condiments to go with main food items.

Breakfast served is a filled 2 inch buttermilk biscuit. Fillings include Canadian bacon (1.4 oz.), sausage (1.4 oz.), and Swiss or American cheese (3/4 oz.) in any combination. A Wuvs special includes 1 egg, cheese slice and Canadian bacon on the biscuit. These items are available all day.

The self-serve salad bar has 25 items. There is a variety of vegetables, real bacon bits and sunflower seeds. The house and blue cheese dressings are without added sugar and have a mayonnaise-buttermilk base. Straight vinegar and oil is available. Lemon wedges may be requested.

The meat for hamburgers is grilled and drained. All burgers are "dressed" to order and served on 4" sesame seed buns. Hamburgers are available in two patty sizes – 1.6 oz. and 4 oz. before cooking weight.

A bowl of chili contains 3.5 oz. meat. Fried chicken, onion rings, and French fries are fresh ingredients cooked in peanut oil.

Unsweetened orange juice, Tab, and fresh brewed ice tea are dieters' favorities.

Wuvs tries to accomodate special requests and does a pretty good job for a fast food restaurant. By choosing the biscuit fillings, burger condiments and "doing your own thing" at the salad bar a person on a modified diet can fare well.

## "PERFECT ENDING"

Baskin Robbins
23 S. State St.
(Village Shopping Center)
Lake Oswego, Oregon

Ice cream can be figured into most diets for a special occasion treat. On the diabetic and most weight loss diets a half cup of ice cream equals 160 calories or 1 bread and two fat exchanges.

Ice cream creations by Paul at the Lake Oswego Baskin Robbins will add a festive touch to any occasion – diet or not. Paul creates solid ice cream cakes for all occasions with ice cream icing! Cake specials can be ordered for holidays, birthdays (for kids they're the greatest) and weddings. Wedding cakes are beautiful tiered creations and arrive packed in dry ice. "Any of the ice cream cakes will be good for an hour out of the ice packing" says the creator.

Special interest is given to people with special requests and for that special occasion everything should be perfect – diet and all! These special dessert creations are sure to be guest pleasers without the slightest hint of diet perfect!

A small amount of buttercream decoration may be used on outer edge but is easily removed from the frozen treat and inside servings and cuts would not have any.

Ice cream pies can be specialty orders without the calorie laden crust and have ice cream borders substituted for the sugar filled fudge sauce edges.

At Christmas try the festive snowball treats with coconut snow and bright candles.

Whatever the occasion Paul will try to accomodate your special request. Since he uses all ice cream in his custom desserts, customers may avoid (and surely not miss) the heavily sugared frosting of most treats.

If requested, Paul can also give the approximate portion size for easier diet calculation.

These very special perfect endings are by special order. For more information call Paul or Pam at 636-7187. Celebrate!

P.S. The average Baskin Robbins scoop of ice cream is a 2-1/2 oz. serving. Enjoy!

# INDEX